Praise for H...

"This book truly is a revelation, remindi ...at the right time - that heroic, courageous people really do exist and that they have wonderful stories to tell. I can't remember the last time I've felt this inspired."

Mike Rosenwald
staff writer, *The Washington Post*

"Tim Wambach has given the world the gift of understanding. His story of this unique friendship is a great lesson on getting past appearances to get to what really matter - heart and soul."

Bill Adams,
Communication Coach, Speaker, and Broadcaster
www.empowertalk.com

"This book is the story of a world-class friendship that won't quit. It's reminder to us all about what really matters most in life."

Steve Siebold CSP
author,speaker

"This book will touch your heart and inspire your soul. It's a true testament of courage, inspiration and friendship and will remind you of the importance of appreciating others."

James Malinchak
Contributing Author to Chicken Soup for the Soul
"America's Hottest Young Speaker"
www.Malinchak.com

"Mike and Tim's story will open your eyes to the world of special needs. Their special bond is an example of two world's gliding together in harmony."

Pat Williams
Senior Vice President of the NBA's Orlando Magic

"There is no glamorous side of having cerebral palsy, but Mike and Tim show that with laughter and perseverance the road can be a little more easily traveled down."
Alison T. Coleman

"*How We Roll* shares the journey of two men learning about life, one was a man with CP the other his aide. It's a great book that tells about friendship and lifes Journey's. Who learnt more? It is hard to say but see how Mike and Tim learned more from each other than a class room could teach."
Robin Pritts, CPA
Author of *From CP to CPA: One Man's Triumph over the disability of Cerebral Palsy*

"I found the book a great inspiration. The story inspires you to want to aim higher in your life and achieve your goals. I have a less severe form of CP, but it doesn't matter if you are disabled or not, this book has some great lessons in how to enjoy life's journey. I would recommend it to anyone. I personally am so pleased to be able to call Tim and Mike my friends, and share in their story. I feel like I have known them all my life."
Susie Bennett, UK
author of *The Sky's the Limit* and the blog LivingwithCerebralPalsy.com

HOW WE ROLL

Earl,   10-2-13

Dude! You are AMAZING! Thank
you for your service! Let us know how
we can help!   847-322-1297

     Keep On Keeping On,

     Tim
     Wambles

HOW WE ROLL

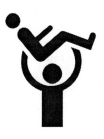

2 friends,
1 wheelchair and a
lifetime of lessons
in perseverance

Tim Wambach

Advantage®

Copyright © 2010 by Tim Wambach

All rights reserved. No part of this book may be used or reproduced in any manner whatsoever without prior written consent of the author, except as provided by the United States of America copyright law.

Published by Advantage, Charleston, South Carolina.
Member of Advantage Media Group.

ADVANTAGE is a registered trademark and the Advantage colophon is a trademark of Advantage Media Group, Inc.

Printed in the United States of America.

ISBN: 978-1-59932-159-2
LCCN: 2010902184

This publication is designed to provide accurate and authoritative information in regard to the subject matter covered. It is sold with the understanding that the publisher is not engaged in rendering legal, accounting, or other professional services. If legal advice or other expert assistance is required, the services of a competent professional person should be sought.

Most Advantage Media Group titles are available at special quantity discounts for bulk purchases for sales promotions, premiums, fundraising, and educational use. Special versions or book excerpts can also be created to fit specific needs.

For more information, please write: Special Markets, Advantage Media Group, P.O. Box 272, Charleston, SC 29402 or call 1.866.775.1696.

Visit us online at **advantagefamily**.com

Dedication

To the Creative Crusader who taught me how to make my limits disappear.

In memory of Jeff Jones and Marty LeBaron

Table of Contents

Acknowledgments

First, I give thanks to my parents, Martin and Letitia. They have been the most supportive parents a son could ask for. I have no idea where I would be without their guidance. They both started their careers as teachers, and they taught me how to be a caring, loving individual. I love you guys so much.

I also thank my grandparents who have all passed on – Alexander and Rosella Wambach and Dr. Stanley and Cecilia Koziol. I'm lucky to have this lineage.

Obviously, I thank Denis and Linda Berkson. I thank them for letting me in their life and trusting me with their sons. Mike and David have been a gift in my life. Without them, my life would have less meaning.

I thank the integral members of Team KOKO – David Kunicki, Dan Joyce, Katie Corboy, Bernadette Elenteny, Bridget Mutter, Renata Johns, Molly Mulcrone and Judy Nowak. Your dedication to this cause has made a tremendous difference in countless lives. I can't tell you enough how much you mean to me.

There are so many people to thank: Here is a list, in no particular order. You have made a difference in Mike's life and mine.

The first person I have to thank is Stacey Dennis. She was my sounding board, best friend and worst critic throughout the creation of this book, and her creative insights are laced throughout its pages. When I needed a push, she was there. When I need a listening ear, she was there. When tension was high, she calmed it. Thanks, babe!

I also thank Dan Walsh, Steve Lesniak, Jason Robinson, Dianne Sroka, Mike's bus drivers Bud, Bill, and Rose, Bonnie Wallace, Mrs. McNish, Mr. Buzard, Dave Tosh, Jan Christensen, John Curtain, Mrs. Daly, Mrs. Fisk, Mrs. Herling, Mrs. Kondiles, Mrs. Linder, Rachel Meyer, Vince Micari, Ms. Molloy, Alex Posner, Mr. Rottman, Jim Schaefer, Tom Leonas, Mrs. Shiner, Officer Ken Smith (Springman), Megan Stambaugh, Andrea Voorhies, Mrs. Walton, LeAnne Hotton, Mr. Kerr, Mr. Eich, John Sullivan, Hector Carabez, Cecile Frydman, Terry Harris, Todd Hansen, Scott McDermott, Kara Bolf, Julie Pielin, Sara Schroeder, Brian Whalen, Kurt Anderson, Mary Zuccarello, Del Kennedy, Debbie Middleton, Alison Guenther, Greg Stolzer, Anita and Jim Descourouez, Chuck Haley, Officer Ken Smith (Glenbrook South), Dan Seeburg, James Kuchienski, Dave Durdov, Liam Gilhooly, Jill Koenig, Gerry Rogers, Joe Novak, Josh Kain, Kendra Ceicita, Cara Johnson, Wendy Blackwell, Kevin Roy, Garrett Farnsworth, Matt Powell, Noel Swan, Lou Vinci, Adam Carroll, Chad Carden, Pat Williams, Adam Witty, Dr. Bernard Brommel, Melanie Pierce, Mitch Rosen, Matt Abbatacola, Chris Rongey, Jeff Corder, Nikki Chuminatto, Todd Ganz, Lauren Kunicki, Sean Tenner, Dan Maynulet, Timmy Maloney, Nish Vartabedian, TJ Royce, Andrew Miller, Teri Szymczak, Eric Edholm, Laura Girolami, Tamika Boyd, Lucy Hernandez, Dawn Moore, Dawn Zeribicki, Corissa Todd, Dr. Mats Gunnars, Tim Brennan, Jeff and Elena Moirano, Christa Loman, Lisa Henschel, Jonathan Keaton, John "Big Johnny" Hartman, Vic and Pam Kunicki, Rita Mueller, Jeff "JAQ" Qaiyum, Ed Wolf, Craig Glicken, Bryan Ogren, Dave and Katalin Ogren, Adie Zuckerman, Jim Dusablon, Steve and Karen Schada, Mark and Anne Mlinar, Richard and Mary Kunicki, Larry Patrick, Mike Maguire, Julie Prato, Jim Shellard, Mark Maranto, Eddie Itkin, The Antonucci Family, Myra Gorman, Leonard Woodson, Farkus—Tony Maguire, Brian Gilliam,

DD and Kevin Coyne, Ryan Fuss, Patti Interrante, Tony Churchill, Lil' Johnny Frisco, Bill Paige, Lars Anderson, Rob Pritts, Sarah Vargo, Jen Knoedl, Stu Mittleman, Mark and Janel Blakely, Don and Ruth Koziol, Len Koziol, Richard Wambach, Tim and Nicole O'Connor, Britt Wambach, Dave and Natasha Felski, Jack and Sue Bringer, Jim and Mary O'Malley, Bob and Debbie Cole, Sue Blacklock, Sharon Kenny, Fr. Greg Sakowicz, Fr. Leo Mahon, and all the St. Mary of the Woods staff.

And let me offer special thanks to anyone who has opened a door for Mike and me.

Foreword
By Denis Berkson, Mike's father

This book is about going forward. It is about looking at what is in your life, pushing it out of your way, moving past it, and continuing with the journey. It is about what you can do when you are moving forward, even as you look back at your experiences. You can gather up all those experiences and put them in a bag and use them in some way. If you can find a way to interpret them, to give them meaning, they will propel you forward to the next step, which is where you are supposed to be. This is a book about doing just that.

Imagine a giant brown bear in the woods, standing on his hind legs, his paws stretching toward the sky. Imagine that the bear is smiling – the biggest smile you have ever seen on any creature, from one side of his face to the other. Now, picture that bear skipping down a path through the woods. Just before he disappears from sight, he turns slowly to wave at you with a big, brown paw, as if to say, "See ya, I'm moving on."

You have just met Tim – or at least, that's how I thought of Tim when I first met him: a big, gentle guy. From our first handshake, I knew he was a man moving forward.

Tim and I met in 2001 at Springman Middle School, where I was interviewing him to be an aide for my son, Mike, who has cerebral palsy. Mike is limited in his arm and leg mobility, and he needs a wheelchair, but his IQ soars off the charts. Little did I know then that the gentleman sitting across from me, that big brown bear with that contagious smile who was in motion 99.9 percent of the time, would become my third son.

Tim and Mike formed a friendship at that middle school, a bond that has continued – that has moved forward – to this day. Each discovered something within the other that connected them. Each discovered in the other something that inspired them. Such was the basis of the friendship you will read about in this book. My son Mike, and Tim, who is my son in spirit, have a great deal in common, and they are truly pals.

The "P" in pal stands for patience. Tim has developed a great patience in the world of special needs. He may operate a little differently than others, and perhaps he has had more frustrations and a few more obstacles, but nonetheless Tim has shown a patience and concern that are truly special in a young man. Mike also exhibits that characteristic of patience. He is patient because things may not happen as quickly or as diligently as he might want them to. He is patient when he has to adapt to his surroundings or to what is done to him. Patience is one of the lifelines keeping Tim and Mike together.

The "A" in pal stands for attitude. Both Tim and Mike have incredible attitudes. Each believes that whether you can or cannot, you are correct. Tim thinks big. Mike thinks bigger. Mike dreams big. Tim dreams bigger. Each looks at the world where there are some dark spots, and they see some light. Where there is a little sadness, they see a whole lot of potential for happy. Whenever it seems something cannot be, that is when each of their faces lights up and says, "It will be. I can do it. We can do it."

And "L" stands for light – as in the words to that old song, "This little light of mine, I'm going to make it shine." Sometimes everybody's light flickers a little, but I think that when that happens to Mike, Tim is there to help get him glowing again – to give him a pep talk and a pat on the back, or maybe just listen. I think the same is true from Mike's point of view. Whenever Tim is getting a little down, perhaps losing his way a little bit, Mike gives him some feedback, some ideas, some advice – or just listens.

What a friendship! Two guys, living in two different worlds. As you read this book, I think you will see that those worlds don't collide but rather glide together. There's Mike, sitting in his wheelchair, tooling this way and that, and there's Tim skipping down the path, going where he has to go. Two men off to see the world. As you read these pages, you are going to see that world, and I think that when you do, you will get a smile on your face, as I do.

You will see that big bear skipping down that forest path, and you will also see a faithful companion coming up quickly to his side. As you watch them go over that hill together, I think that your face and your heart will smile. And perhaps you, too, will feel inspired – inspired to move forward.

Denis is the author of *10 Demandments of Creativity – Parents Edition.*

Chapter 1

"Everything Happens for a Reason"

"A consistent soul believes in destiny, a capricious one in chance."
Benjamin Disraeli

This is the story of how Mike and I met, grew together, and taught each other from our separate worlds. Mike taught me patience, strength and perseverance by way of humor. I taught Mike…well, I suggest you read on to find out. First, let me introduce you to Mike. I know he will move you, as he has moved me. Here's Mike's story, in his own words:

David popped out first, slick as a whistle with a glistening bald head and screeching like a gossiping teenage girl. The nurse shushed him to no avail, wrapped the writhing newborn in blankets, and set him aside to grab me, Mike. She turned to find the doctor's arms still outstretched, awaiting my arrival, and joined him in coaxing my mom to push. Fashionably late and cute as a button, I made my grand entrance without a solitary whimper. It was February 4, 1989.

The nurse swaddled me in blankets as I smiled my signature devilish grin – one that I still flaunt whilst outsmarting David or seducing the ladies. David and I were adorable little babies, and we giggled obligingly as various relatives wielded squeaky toys while making indecipherable sounds. My show-off brother waved his chubby little arms about, reaching for the stuffed clown or toy car. I did not. At three months, David flaunted his mad mobile skills, rolling across the room and laughing. I did not.

So Mom and I visited the doctor, a tall skinny man with a long nose that loomed over a tiny, unkempt mustache. He never smiled, and he smelt of Bengay and Aqua Velva, a blend I do not recommend as cologne. He cleared his throat, crossed his arms, and in a monotone voice he said: "I regret to inform you that Mike has cerebral palsy, in all likelihood due to lack of oxygen in the birth canal during labor. He will never speak, walk or think like a normal child."

My parents understood and accepted the weight of the circum-stance, yet they refused to believe the extent of the doctor's predictions. Call it denial. I like to call it hope.

Within three years, I finally won at a game of sibling rivalry—I spoke more words than my able-bodied brother. Despite my limited mobility, my energetic mind absorbed the words and occurrences that enveloped me, and I spoke with conviction. My mom and I returned to that foul-smelling doctor, and at her instruction, I said to him: "Quit your day job." He did not respond.

Eight years after that doctor's visit, I entered the sixth grade. With the assistance of an aide, I got to and from school, completed my assignments via dictation, and attended sixth-grade classes alongside my biped peers. I can read; however, because focal dystonia causes contractions of the muscles around my eyes, it takes me half an hour to read a paragraph. It's tiresome, and I often answered test questions wrong when I rushed an answer after concentrating so long and hard on reading the question. In the interest of time (and my sanity), my aide assisted me with assignments, tests and quizzes by reading the questions and recording my responses. When test taking time arrived, my aide and I left the classroom so as not to disrupt the class (or give away answers). One day, after I had confidently aced a vocabulary quiz, my teacher requested that I stay after class.

"Mike, you were the only student who got a 100 percent on the quiz yesterday." I smiled and awaited her praise. "I'm going to ask you a question," she continued, "and I want you to answer honestly, OK?" She spoke in a slow, robotic tone.

"Yes," I replied.

"Did you have help?"

"Help?"

Then I understood. She was bewildered at how I could have excelled. No disabled student had ever done so before, she explained: Had I cheated?

"No!" I firmly replied. I looked at my aide. "Let's roll," I said, wishing I could storm out and slam the door.

At first, I felt angry. I felt insulted. It was then that I transformed my anger into sympathy. I felt sorry for those who harbor such ignorance. Thereafter, this common misconception that there is a direct and concrete link between physical disability and mental disability ceased to shock or anger me. I now simply laugh at its idiocy.

I'm reminded of the expression "so close and yet so far." My body may not work in the able-bodied world, but my mind does. In the same way a blind man's sense of hearing is enhanced, my mind is sharp. I have a thirst for knowledge. I have ideas. I have goals.

Overall, I am very similar to everyone else — the one difference being that my lack of physicality affects my daily life. I cannot write or type. I cannot brush my own teeth. I cannot feed myself. I cannot use the toilet. I simply cannot perform many of the little, everyday functions that so many take for granted.

Throughout my schooling, the emphasis on special education often bothered me. I understood the need for special education; however, teachers and administrators often determined an education plan without considering the student's specific needs, strengths and weaknesses. I felt that my voice went unheard and that my challenges to standard procedures were viewed as pride-driven and defiant.

For example, I cannot use a voice activated computer because I have a speech impediment caused by difficulty with breath control. Nonetheless, every year, my "Individual Education Plan" insisted the technology had improved. Every year, I tried, and on a good day I could complete a sentence in an hour. "Give it another shot," the teachers said. I was frustrated not because they pushed the device but rather because no one listened to me. The adults were not voice activated. They so passionately wanted the device to work that they ignored the fact that it simply did not work for me.

Let's consider the word "independent." It is defined as "not requiring or relying on something else or someone else." In a perfect world, I would adhere to that as best I could. But I can't. So I've created my own definition: "thoughts and choices not requiring or relying on outside influences." I make my own decisions, I create my own opinions, and I have ownership of my thoughts, and I am therefore independent. Unfortunately, those who can control their extremities do not necessarily understand my definition. "You should use a power chair," they say. "It will make you independent. You will feel empowered! You can go places! Do whatever you want!"

I often suspect that the physically handicapped feel cornered, or perhaps, bullied into the belief that every modification designed for the physically disabled is 100 percent right for them. I don't believe that. Certainly, a power wheelchair would give me the ability to move freely, but at what cost? The effort spent to extend my arm and control the joystick exhausted me to the point that I did not want to do anything else. I know what you are thinking. Practice makes perfect, right? But I cannot open a door. I cannot glance at the back of a DVD box or book jacket. I cannot operate a computer. I cannot pick up a pencil. The point is: I still need someone else to do everything for me. So what would a power chair truly empower me to do?

Everyone is entitled to an opinion, and I certainly have a few. But I do not force my opinions on others. I do not tell an overweight man to choose a salad over pizza. I do not tell a woman on the street to consider a thong when her panty line is showing. (I can't help but notice; it's in my direct line of sight.) I do not tell a healthy teenager that I see at the mall to stop smoking and cut his ridiculously long, messy hair. I do not tell bored-looking couples what new sexual positions to try.

Now, these examples may seem extreme and inappropriate, but so is someone telling me what chair to use. I am very aware of what I can't do. I would rather accept what I cannot do and focus on what I can do.

Fear not. I may have problems. But I have no complaints. I find ways to cope. My sharp sense of humor allows me to shrug off some of the not-so-pleasant aspects of my disability. I never dwell on my limita-

tions. Focusing on my disability will not make my legs move or my back straighten.

Instead, I ponder unlimited possibilities. I aspire to direct films, and I will. When I feel doubt or depression beginning to creep in, I watch a movie. For as long as I can remember, Dad and I went to the movies every Saturday. Some might say I have an interesting taste in film. My cinematic preferences range from the crude and quirky to violent, Tarentino-esque films. I like violence. I like weirdness. I like darkness.

I once commented to my mom: "If people knew my taste in movies and didn't know me, they would consider me crazy." She replied, "Even people who know you think you're crazy, my dear."

But a little crazy is good. And a lot of the good kind of crazy came into my life the year after I almost lost my faith in people because of a teacher's ignorance.

And there you have it, straight from Mike—and I'm proud to have been the bearer of the good kind of craziness that made his life, and mine, better forever.

I was twenty-six years old, living with my parents in Niles, Ill., and in major debt—not quite the life I'd envisioned. This came after the failure of a seminar that I had single-handedly promoted and financed.

The seminar, geared toward teens, had offered the secrets to success. How ironic. Ten thousand dollars later, with my dream of professional speaking fading into the distance, I hit bottom. Then, my girlfriend ended our two-year relationship with the infamous "it's not you, it's me" excuse.

Without direction and utterly lost, I settled for a job at a GNC nutrition store. My pimply-faced boss, four years my junior – and, adding insult to injury, a Green Bay Packers fan – drove me crazy. I disliked the job immensely.

I endured by continually reminding myself that everything happens for a reason. That reason revealed itself shortly thereafter.

During my commute to GNC, I passed School District 34's administration office in Glenview. On a whim, I stopped by one day before work and applied for a substitute teaching position. Again, that wasn't my ideal job, but I felt I'd rather teach pimply-faced kids than be bossed around by one. I'd always enjoyed working with children and young adults, having served as a youth minister and special education camp leader during college.

In response to my application, a district administrator asked if I would be interested in working one-on-one with an eighth-grade girl who had cerebral palsy. The job meant a regular schedule, benefits, and a degree of stability that I hadn't had in months. I interviewed with Dan Walsh, head of student services at Springman Middle School. After going through four aides in five months, Dan would have settled for anyone with a pulse who would commit until the end of the year. I was over-qualified.

I met Rachel the next Monday. Everyone seemed impressed with how well I worked with Rachel, which confused me a little. Something distinguished me from my predecessors. I comforted Rachel. I made her giggle with my silly antics. I simply cared.

If not for my desperate situation, I might not have taken that $9 per hour job. To be honest, I felt somewhat inferior to my friends who had steady, high-income careers and their own homes. But again, there's always a reason.

At the end of the school year, as Rachel's graduation neared, Dan asked me to work with an incoming seventh grader the following year. I hesitated at first. I feared becoming comfortable in a job that I enjoyed but that would not beget my ultimate goals. I did not want to lose sight of my dream of professional speaking and authorship.

"Just meet Denis, the boy's father," Dan implored. I conceded.

A few days later, I walked into Dan's office to find a stocky, burly man with a thick mustache and an ear piercing. He approached me with a big smile and an outstretched hand. After the customary small talk, Denis told me about his son, Mike.

"Mike is the coolest kid ever," he said. He described Mike's quick wit, extraordinary intelligence, and movie mania.

"And David, Mike's twin, he's the second coolest kid ever." Denis chuckled. "David is a special soul – an old soul. He and Mike are best friends." Denis told me that he and his wife, Linda, couldn't do without David, who understood the care and attention that Mike needed and the sacrifices required by all. "He always helps and never complains."

Everyone in the family, he said, depended on one another. When Linda takes Mike to therapy, he explained, David helps transfer Mike in and out of the van. On returning home, they change Mike, a task that David never tries to avoid. "Meanwhile, I pick up a movie and dinner on my way home from work," Denis said, "and I often have to stop at more than one place if Mike wants pancakes and David, a slice of pizza."

He looked deeply into my eyes. "You see, Tim, Mike isn't the only one with CP. We all have cerebral palsy." His words touched me, and I offered to work with Mike over the summer.

Chapter 2

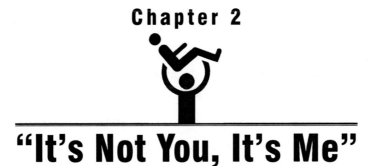

"It's Not You, It's Me"

"You can't live a perfect day without doing something for
someone who will never be able to repay you."
Coach John Wooden

Mike and David were completing sixth grade at Pleasant Ridge
School and were going to be the hosts of a talent show titled
"Crouching Students, Hidden Talents."

"Mike came up with the title!" Denis exclaimed with pride.
Wow, creative! I thought, already impressed. I couldn't wait to meet the
Berkson brothers.

On the day of the show, I found a seat near the back of the packed,
flamboyantly decorated auditorium. Denis noticed me and shot me a
wave and big smile as the lights dimmed in anticipation of the hosts'
entrance.

A teacher wheeled Mike out first. Mike's words were slow and
mildly distorted, but audible: "Welcome to Crouching Students,
Hidden Talents. My brother and co-host, David, is running a little

late. While we await his arrival, I will advise you, my fellow peers, of five things you never want to try while naked."

He cleared his throat. "Five, fry bacon. Four, clear a patch of poison ivy. Three, bathe a cat. Two, operate a blowtorch. And the number one thing you should never do naked: host a talent show for kids."

David's head peeked out from behind the curtain. "What was that last one, Mike?" David extended his bare leg from behind the makeshift curtain, as the audience gasped. He revealed himself, fully clothed in a Bears T-shirt and shorts. The audience laughed and cheered.

Stunned, I did neither. Mike and David were identical, down to their matching crew cuts and black-rimmed glasses. Neither Dan nor Denis had mentioned that Mike and David were *identical* twins. A flurry of thoughts ran through my mind: How difficult that must be for Mike, to have an exact CP-free replica of himself – to watch his healthy duplicate walk, run, and go out with friends. And David must feel so guilty, as the one without cerebral palsy.

I quieted my mind as the show began, giving the boys my complete attention. I enjoyed the dynamic between the two. I laughed until I cried, overwhelmed by this marvel unfolding before me – a young boy with cerebral palsy and a killer sense of humor, his equally hilarious identical brother who played off him so fluidly, and a wheelchair that disappeared before my eyes as I began to see Mike as a quick-witted 12-year-old, not a boy with a disability.

Afterward, I met the gang – Mike's mom, Linda; his teachers; his aide; and finally, Mike and David. We walked outside, greeted by humidity and elongated daylight – the first indications of summer in Chicago. "Great job, guys! That was awesome!" I impulsively rubbed

Mike's head, an act that became my customary display of affection. He smiled.

"Here comes Dad!" David exclaimed. Denis drove up in a hot set of wheels—a big, gray conversion van.

"C'mon Tim," Denis said. "We're going to Blockbuster, then home for a little 'R&R'—R-rated movie and relaxation. And you're coming with us."

Denis instructed me on how to load Mike into the van. Denis opened the side door and pressed a button, prompting a lift to automatically extend and lower. He pushed Mike on, and then secured the chair to the lift. Once the lift was up, we pushed his chair into the van. Securing his chair required linking a small bolt on the bottom of the chair to a small metal lock on the van floor. This required great precision and patience. Denis and I had to pull the chair in and out of the van a few times before the bolt finally snapped into the lock.

"You'd think after twelve years my aim would be better," Denis joked, patting my back.

David sat behind Mike, and I joined Denis in the front, while Linda drove home separately. Mike and David chatted about their brilliant performance as I looked from one to the other, still mesmerized by their resemblance—dark hair, glasses, blue eyes, big smile, and long, skinny legs.

Mike entered the video store with a determined look. He had a mission—to find a movie ridden with crude humor. He selected *Deuce Bigalow: Male Gigolo*. Denis looked at me and shrugged. "It's what he likes."

Shortly before dark, we arrived at the Berkson home, a single-level ranch home complete with basketball hoop in the driveway and abandoned bike on the lawn. David ran in first, hurried by the call of nature, followed by Mike, Denis and me. I closed the door, and when I turned back to the foyer, something small darted toward my eyes. I ducked, almost stumbling forward, enveloped by the uproarious laughter of Denis, Mike and Linda. I looked around, confused.

"That's just a little *annoying*," Mike said sarcastically.

"*Augie*," Denis corrected promptly. "Sorry, Tim, every now and then we like to let the birds out. Tweet…tweet tweet tweet."

"Dad, please," Mike said, embarrassed by his father's lame attempt at pop culture word play. "Put the dogs back in, along with your bad jokes. OK, Dad?" I laughed, my heart rate decelerating.

"Isn't it pronounced *dawgs*?"

Mike sighed. "I wish I could roll my eyes right now."

"What'd I miss?" David asked when he returned from the bathroom.

"Augie tried to kill Tim," Mike replied.

"Doesn't surprise me."

"C'mon in. Make yourself at home," Denis said as he cajoled Augie to his palm and returned him to a cage in the living room. I followed him into the living room and noticed a second bird in the cage. The two resembled miniature parrots and chirped piercingly loud.

"They're called lovebirds," Denis said. "Say *hello*…say *hello*…." Denis tapped the cage but elicited only repeated chirps. He shrugged. "They're still learning."

Their home, adorned with family portraits and candid photos and a bowl of candy on every table, felt warm and welcoming. The furniture was spread out, allowing plenty of room for maneuvering Mike.

"You have a lovely home," I said.

"Thank you," Linda replied.

While Denis and Linda got snacks together and David started the movie, Mike took me to his room and excitedly showed me his film collection, with such titles as *Pulp Fiction, Friday, Nightmare on Elm Street,* and *The Blues Brothers.* His walls were covered with posters of rappers, but few whom I recognized.

"Most kids in my school like 50 Cent, Ja Rule, and those sorta rappers," he said. "That's pop rap and manufactured anger. I prefer less mainstream artists like Dr. Dre, Ice-T and Tech 9. Real rap artists transform their struggles into art. It resonates with me." I was as captivated by Mike's fascination with rap as I was with his taste in movies.

"You didn't expect me to like rap, did you?"

"Mike, from the moment you took that stage, I learned not to have any expectations. I have a feeling you will never cease to shock and amaze."

He smiled. "You have no idea." I didn't.

"We're ready!" David shouted.

Mike and I returned to the living room, and I wheeled him to the center of the room at Linda's instruction. She attached a tray to his chair, placed a book in front of him and the remote control atop the book. This enabled him to navigate the remote control. He looked at me. "It's the only thing I can physically control on my own," he said.

I sat on the floor next to him, and observed as he raised his hand over the remote, struggled to steady his fingers, and pressed play. A pang of guilt shot through me – something I would feel again and again as I got to know Mike. I realized how many little things I took for granted.

Later that night, as Denis drove me back to my car at the school, he asked with a hint of sarcasm, "So, has the crazy Berkson clan scared you off, or are you still interested in working with Mike?"

"Denis, I thrive on crazy. I'm thrilled to work with Mike." With that, we set up a first "man-date" for Mike and me.

At Mike's request, our first adventure took us to the Northbrook Court Mall. For mindless trivia fanatics, the *Weird Science* film scene where Anthony Michael Hall gets doused by a Slurpee was filmed there. On the way, with the windows down and a warm breeze on our faces, we listened to loud rap music while I flaunted my crazy car-dancing moves, gyrating my shoulders and pumping my fists (at red lights, of course). People stopped and stared, pointed and laughed. I didn't care. Mike loved it.

As I wheeled Mike through the mall, in and out of almost every store, I was taken aback by the frequent stares and uncomfortable glances. Children, prompted by their innate, innocent curiosity, stared and pointed.

"Mommy, what's the matter with him?" one child asked. The mother snatched the child's outstretched hand. "It's not polite to stare and point," she scolded.

Some adults, without the excuse of infancy, stared at Mike with a countenance of disapproval or fleetingly averted their eyes, clearly discomforted. Others, the ones I admire, simply smiled and nodded without regard for the wheelchair or Mike's awkward posture.

I felt immense sympathy not only for Mike but also for those who beheld him. Somehow we are preconditioned, perhaps by parents who chide our curiosity, to judge appearances. If only that mom would have smiled and told her pointing child, "Yes, dear, that boy has a blue shirt just like yours," how different an impression she'd have made. I felt sorry for those people because they missed out on the remarkably talented person who is Mike.

Mike interrupted my thoughts. "I have a hankering for Taco Bell," he said.

Hankering? I thought. *What are you, ninety?* I would soon find myself astonished at Mike's expressiveness and expansive vocabulary. I would be learning a new word almost every day.

I had never fed Mike before, and he ever so kindly introduced me to the experience with a beef MexiMelt and a soft taco. We began with the soft taco. I held it to Mike's mouth, and he took a big bite. The contents spewed everywhere. Mike's T-shirt sustained significant wounds from the explosion of beef, cheese, onions and lettuce. After five big bites, the taco was obliterated. The debris covered Mike, my hands, the wheelchair, the table.

I must have looked discouraged. Mike burst out laughing.

"What?"

"It's all right, Tim. It's not you, it's me."

"I've heard that before."

"Hey," he said. "Don't cry over spilled Taco Bell."

Now, for those who might have found themselves staring at such a sight, and perhaps judging, I propose a challenge. Ask a friend to tie your hands behind your back and attempt to feed you a soft taco, a hamburger, or a slice of deep dish pizza. Make sure your friend can be trusted to untie you afterward, and never again take your taco-eating ability for granted.

A few days later, Mike, David and I were off to the movies to see *Lara Croft: Tomb Raider*. With rap music blaring and car-dancing in action, Mike suddenly exclaimed, "Angelina Jolie! Yum…."

Mike may use a wheelchair, but he's still a 12–year-old boy filled with hormones, I thought with a smile.

Today's menu consisted of extra-buttery popcorn and soda – grub much easier to contend with, though my fingers got butter-soaked and sticky. We found a handicapped-accessible area to sit, and then proceeded to watch Angelina strut around in a tight little outfit for two hours, much to Mike's satisfaction.

When I dropped the boys off at their home, David challenged me to an NBA Live 2001 game on their PlayStation.

"Are you sure?" I asked.

"I can take you," he replied confidently.

Thus began an epic battle on the hardwood. David did not stand a chance. I floated across the court, blocking shots, hitting threes and jammin' dunks the way MJ did in the late '80s. I brought my A-game to the court, together with my ruthless smack talk. "Nice try, Marbury! Maybe you should have stayed at Georgia Tech for your sophomore year!"

Despite David's valiant attempt, his efforts were futile. "I'm sorry you have to witness this," I told Mike. "In a little bit, you will be called to identify the body, 'cause Davey's getting killed!" I celebrated my victory – or should I say I flaunted my victory. David looked discouraged.

"Davey, I may be in my late twenties, but I can still play some video games. I got experience on you, novice."

"Looks like you met your match, bro!" Mike teased. David was still shocked by the butt-whopping he had just been served.

As Mike and Denis walked me out, David bear-hugged Denis from behind, startling his dad. Denis responded by poking him, and the two began exchanging jabs and laughing. I came to Denis' rescue, grabbing David by the waist and wrestling him to the floor. Denis slammed his hand on the carpet. "One, two, three, you're out! The winner and champion is Timmy Wambach!" Denis exclaimed. I jumped up like Rocky and hit the Berksons with my best Balboa impression. "I just want to say one thing. Yo Adrian, I did it!"

Driving home that night, I felt a sense of peace. In such a short time, I'd become a part of the Berkson clan. Life has a way of giving us what we need most. I had needed stability and a sense of contribution. Back in January, I'd felt like a ship without a rudder, sail or wind – and now the missing pieces were coming together. My positive outlook began to resurface.

Chapter 3

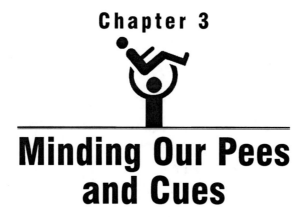

Minding Our Pees and Cues

"Laughter is the shortest distance between two people."
Victor Borge

That September, I was attending a seminar in Hawaii so I could not start working with Mike at the beginning of the school year. In my absence, Dan, the head of student services, hired a registered nurse named Cindy to serve as Mike's aide. Upon my return to Illinois, Dan wanted me at Springman. Although he did not have a specific position for me, he considered me an asset and requested that I assist wherever needed. My first assignment was to shadow a potentially hostile student who had threatened one of his peers.

During times when that student was in class, Cindy asked that I help her with Mike's bathroom visits. I also helped with his "stander" time – a stander is an instrument that allows people like Mike to stretch their limbs a couple times a day. I found my shadowing responsibility rather dull, so the intermittent breaks were the highlight of my day – even the bathroom breaks.

I can't imagine how utterly uncomfortable it must have been for Mike to be transferred to a changing table by Cindy and me and to be assisted with something so private. I tried to break the tension by acting foolish. I spoke in silly voices, spouted out popular movie quotes, and made mindless jokes—anything to take Mike's mind off the situation.

Sometimes I broke into my Howard Cosell imitation when we would lay Mike onto the table: "Down goes Frazier, down goes Frazier!" Or I imitated the cowardly lion, "Put 'em up, put 'em up, I will beat you with one paw tied behind my back."

And as my pièce de résistance, I recreated the barber shop scene from *Coming to America*. "He beat Joe Louis's ass." "That's true, that's true, he did whoop him." "His momma calls him Cassius. I am going to call him Cassius." "Joe Louis was one hundred thirty-seven years old." "Every time someone brings up Joe Louis, some white guy has to bring up Rocky Marciano … Rocky Marciano. Rocky Marciano."

The skits weren't stellar by any means, but they made Mike smile and redirected his focus. After a while, I looked forward to bathroom breaks, a.k.a. "performance time." Sometimes while watching TV or a movie, I would jot down funny lines. I enjoyed Mike's laughter prompted by my crazy silliness. We developed a bond, a sense of trust. As the task of changing Mike became more routine, I paid less attention to the process and more to making Mike chuckle. Mike felt comfortable with me, and we began to take unspoken cues from each other, all the while laughing and firing Seinfeld quotes back and forth.

"She had man hands."

"This fruit is sub par."

"Amazing. I drive them to lesbianism, and he brings 'em back!"

"And you want to be my latex salesman."

"He's not a Nazi. He just happens to be a little eccentric. Most geniuses are."

"I need the secure packaging of Jockeys. My boys need a house!"

"It's the financial equivalent of a complete rectal examination."

"Mansiere … That's right. A brassiere for a man."

"I slipped and fell on Jerry's head. We've been close ever since."

One day, as Cindy attempted to lift Mike without assistance, she suffered a hernia. She could not return to work until her doctor gave her clearance. I enthusiastically stepped in. I loved every minute of working with Mike, even though I was twenty-eight years old and back in seventh grade. Mike nicknamed me Billy Madison.

"Pay attention, Billy Boy," Mike said on my first day. "You might learn a little something." He smiled that classic sly little smile. *Smartass*, I thought.

I decided to help him with his bathroom visits without assistance. Mike didn't mind. "As long as you don't drop me."

"I won't. I promise."

"I've heard that before." Apparently Denis had dropped him more than once.

"No wonder you have such a lumpy head," I teased.

"Hardy-har-har."

Mike got me back for that joke a few days later, unintentionally of course. During one such bathroom visit, we were greeted by a ghastly scent. It smelled like road kill. The smell seeped out from the drain and enveloped the room.

"Man, can you smell that?" I asked.

"How can you not? My nostrils hurt."

I changed Mike quickly. As I removed his diaper, the stench from the drain worsened, and my face turned white—the look of imminent vomiting.

Suddenly Mike started shaking uncontrollably. I quickly grasped him and held on, afraid he might fall. Fear shot through me. "Mike, what's wrong?!" It was then that I realized he was laughing wildly.

Without warning, a projectile of yellow liquid shot in my direction. Mike, still in his fit of laughter, was completely unaware. I backed up against the wall, hoping he could not project that far. He could. My shirt, shorts and arms were soaked.

When Mike noticed his urine-drenched aide, his laughter came to a screeching halt, as did his robust, seemingly unending stream. We looked at each other in silence, then abruptly ripped into uncontrollable laughter. And Mike wasn't finished. The new round of hilarity triggered yet another projectile stream of urine. I just kept on laughing.

After regaining control, I replaced Mike's diaper. "I don't know why I'm putting this on," I told him. "You won't need one for another two weeks!" I washed my hands while Mike apologized profusely.

"Dude, don't apologize. That was the best laugh I've had in months. Maybe years. And, on the even-brighter side, I get to go home for a bit, to shower and change."

We've been close ever since.

Chapter 4

Elevator Wars

"Life is what we make it. Always has been, always will be."
Grandma Moses

Mike had been talking about the upcoming release of *Star Wars: Episode II* for weeks, so I decided to take him and David to see it. As Mike and I made our way to his first class, he smiled and sheepishly inquired, "Do you know what's coming out this weekend?"

"I know. You've mentioned it nine thousand times. *Star Wars: Episode II* … George Lucas … blah, blah, blah."

I tried to conceal my enthusiasm. I, too, couldn't wait to see the movie. When I was a kid, the only thing I loved more than *Star Wars* was baseball (and my parents, I suppose). When *Return of the Jedi* came out, almost every show sold out immediately, and my dad took me at 7 a.m. on a Sunday.

"Mike, I have a great idea for the weekend."

"What?!" he exclaimed.

"What do you say we spend Saturday at the library and research butterflies?"

"Um…no," he replied, frustration smeared across his face.

"OK. How about we drive to Bloomington, Indiana, and eat Burmese food? It's the only Burmese restaurant in the Midwest."

"Tim!" I loved watching him squirm.

"No? Well, I suppose we could go to the movies. There's a new chick flick coming out this weekend. Something with Julia Roberts…." Mike's face turned red, and I decided to put him out of his misery. "Or we could see *Star Wars*. I mean … if you want to."

His eyes widened as he smiled from ear to ear. "That would be awesome!"

Mike noticed his brother in the distance and shouted, "David! Tim's taking us to see *Star Wars* on Saturday!"

He smiled and, in typical David fashion, said, "Kewl."

I played softball that Friday night and decided to pick up the tickets on my way home.

"Three tickets for *Star Wars: Episode II* at 11:30 a.m., please."

"Sorry pal," replied the ticket agent. "It's sold out."

My stomach dropped. Mike would be devastated. He'd been looking forward to it all week. I heard the ticket agent laughing and looked at him angrily.

"Sorry, man, I was just joking around. Working these late shifts gets a little boring. I try to have a little fun every now and then."

Immense relief washed over me as he handed me the tickets. "Thanks, man. That was a good one."

The next morning, the Berkson brothers were all smiles as we drove to the theater, car-dancing all the way. David began parading his moves, and Mike bobbed his head and moved his arms as best he could. When we walked into the theater, I said rather loudly, "Son of a bitch."

David and Mike were startled at first, then chuckled. "What's wrong?" David asked.

I motioned toward the elevator. "Out of order," a sign read.

"Uh-oh," David said, his voice laced with disappointment. I approached one of the ushers, a teenager blowing gum and humming a Britney Spears song, and she informed me that the elevator would be fixed within the hour.

"That's not good enough," I replied. "We have tickets for the 11:30 show, and we have someone in a wheelchair here!"

"Sorry," she replied, and she resumed chewing and humming.

I thought for a moment, then looked at David and Mike.

"Mike, we will have to call on 'the force.' I have an idea, if you're game."

"What is it?" the boys asked in unison.

"Well, David, I'll need your help. I will carry the wheelchair up the stairs while you hold Mike. Then, I will come down the stairs and carry Mike back to the chair."

"Really?" asked David. "Do you think you can?"

"I don't think I can. I know I can." I channeled Yoda and said, "Always with you, what cannot be done. You must unlearn, what you have learned."

David rolled his eyes and nodded. "OK."

We executed the plan perfectly, amid a few stares and murmurs. I carried the cumbersome wheelchair up the stairs, then returned to relieve David, hoisting Mike over my shoulder.

"Like the view?" I teased, my butt in his face and his in mine.

"I've seen better. You like yours?"

I began the ascent with caution. It was a balancing act, and Mike became heavier with every step. Upon reaching the top, I placed Mike in his chair and groaned loudly, exhausted.

"Thanks for not farting," Mike joked.

Another usher, this one a twentysomething boy with long hair and four ear piercings, approached me. "You know, you really shouldn't have done that. You guys could've gotten hurt."

"Well, if your elevator worked, I wouldn't have had to!" I shouted. "I didn't do it for kicks."

"It's not our fault the elevator is broken."

"It's not Mike's fault, either. Mike wants to see this movie, and I refuse to let your theater's ineptitude ruin it. And the elevator better work within the hour, as promised. Otherwise, your theater will hear from our lawyer."

The boy cleared his throat, and in a shaky tone replied, "Enjoy the movie." He walked away. Quickly.

After the movie, the elevators were working. No need to call Jackie Chiles.

As summer approached, Mike and I had a *hankering* for something different. We would go to the mall, of course, and to our share of movies, but we longed for more adventure. Mike and I scoured the

Internet in search of ideas, and, on the Northwestern University website, an advertisement for a 9/11 exhibit caught our eyes.

"What do you think, Mike?"

"Yeah. That would be cool."

At that moment, Denis entered. "Do you guys want to go swimming at the Jones' pool this summer?"

"How about it?" I asked Mike excitedly.

"I am not much of a swimmer," Mike admitted.

"Really? I had you pegged for a Mark Spitz."

"Sorry, I forgot I was dealing with Ar-NALD. You just want to show off your hot bod in a Speedo." Mike often teased me about my affinity for hitting the gym.

"Yeah baby," I replied, patting my stomach. Unfortunately, I also had an affinity for hitting the bar after softball games, so I was never in tiptop shape.

Two weeks later, Mike and I were off to Evanston for the 9/11 exhibit. We were curious to see how the historical events would be portrayed. I parked, unloaded Mike, and proceeded toward the building – the wrong building, as it turned out. I asked a few passersby, some of them students, others faculty. All seemed confused. One after another, they replied, "Sorry, I can't help you."

Mike looked discouraged. I whispered, "Come on, what did you expect? If it were easy, it wouldn't happen to us. Right?"

"Let's just hope we don't experience *Elevator Wars: Episode II*."

Amen to that, I thought. Traversing any landscape with a wheelchair, be it a school or a movie theater, is a challenge. There are no easy routes. I was still adapting, but it was Mike's reality. He always took it in stride, and with a grain of sarcasm. Our similar go-with-the-flow attitudes strengthened our bond. As one of my high school teachers, Dan Seeburg, often said, "Improvise, adapt, overcome." That became our motto.

Finally, with the assistance of a maintenance man, we located the building that housed the exhibit. "It's on the second floor," he said. "Elevators are that way." He pointed down a long corridor. By the time we reached the end, sweat dripped from my brow.

"Is it raining?" Mike teased, a couple drops of sweat bouncing off his head.

"Ha. Ha." I dried my face with my shirt. "I guess they don't believe in air conditioning."

"Um," Mike said, "they don't believe in elevators either."

I looked up. "What the heck is this?" The "elevator" was a small metal cage without how-to instructions. Improvise, adapt, overcome. I wheeled Mike in, squeezed in next to him, and pulled the cage door shut.

"Now what?" Mike shook wildly, attempting to restrain his laughter. "Thank god you're sitting down and clothed," I told him. "I'm protected against projectile urination." With that, his laughter escaped.

"Tim, this looks like the trash compactor from *Star Wars*, when Luke Skywalker and Han Solo are in that slop and that thing is trying to kill them as the walls come caving in."

"OK, Obi-Wan, how the heck do we get this thing up?"

"Try that button over there," Mike said, attempting to point.

"Where?" I tried to follow his hands, but he jerked left, then right.

"Right there," he urged. Pointing proved fruitless. He couldn't steady his arm long enough for my eyes to follow. He sighed. "Look down and to the left. See it?"

"Got it." My finger hovered hesitantly over the button. "Dude, if we get crushed, how will I explain it to your parents?" Mike laughed. I pushed. Nothing happened. I pushed again. Still nothing. All of a sudden, a loud buzzing noise sounded, startling Mike and me, and the trash compactor began its dreadfully slow ascent.

"Are we there yet?"

"No," I replied.

"How about now?"

"Shut up." I prayed we wouldn't get stuck.

The compactor came to an abrupt halt. "Hallelujah!" I exclaimed. I opened the door. We faced another long – this time, cold – corridor. "Air conditioning," I said. "That's a good sign." Unfortunately, it was not.

The corridor led to a large lobby with a small desk where a middle-aged woman sat engrossed in the latest issue of *People*. "Excuse me, can you direct us to the 9/11 exhibit?"

"Oh, I'm so sorry," she replied. "The opening of the exhibit has been delayed."

I restrained my frustration. "The website clearly states that the exhibit starts today," I protested.

"I'm so sorry," she repeated. "The students aren't ready yet. Have a nice day." She returned to her stimulating reading material.

I looked at Mike. "Sorry, little man, looks like we struck out. I should have called first."

"No worries, Tim," he said, starting to laugh. "Now we get to ride the trash compactor again!"

Next on the adventure reel – swimming at the Joneses. The Joneses' son, Jeff, was inflicted with cerebral palsy more severely than Mike.

When I met Mike, I was unaware of the complexities of CP and how it affects different people in different ways. Over time, I learned. Here's the Cliff's Notes version: Cerebral palsy is an umbrella term covering a group of non-progressive conditions that result in physical handicaps. Experts believe the condition involves connections between the cortex and other parts of the brain such as the cerebellum. Palsy means "disorder of movement." CP is generally categorized into three types—spastic; *athetoid, also known as dyskinetic; and mixed.* Spastic CP refers to excessive muscle tone or tightness. Athetoid CP involves slow, uncontrolled body movements and low muscle tone that makes it hard to sit straight and walk. Mixed CP is a combination of the two—some muscles are too tight, and others are too loose, creating a mix of stiffness and involuntary movements. Also, there are different ways that CP affects the body—diplegia, hemiplegia, and quadriplegia. Diplegia only affects the legs; hemiplegia affects one half of the body, such as the right arm and right leg; and quadriplegia affects both arms and legs and, in some instances, the facial muscles and torso.

Mike and Jeff got the CP trifecta—mixed quadriplegia. Unfortunately, unlike Mike, Jeff's quadriplegia extended to his facial muscles. He could not move his arms and legs, nor could he speak. While there was a lot of life behind his eyes, he could not express it. That is the real tragedy of this condition—it constricts not only mobility, but the ability to communicate as well. You cannot accurately tell your caregiver what you want or need.

Unless you must endure CP yourself, or care for somebody who does, it is impossible to understand. I am still perplexed by it. I see it as a contradiction of philosophies, one that I find hard to explain. Just because someone is in a wheelchair, or cannot communicate effectively, does not mean he needs your help – even if he does need some type of help. You want to treat people with disabilities like everyone else, even though they are not like everyone else and in some ways do require "special" care. But at the same time, they are more capable than you might think, which makes them more like everyone else.

I know, that's a mouthful. But that's how I see it, as convoluted as it may sound.

Back to the story: The Joneses installed a swimming pool to allow Jeff a more enjoyable way of relaxing his muscles.

At first Mike was hesitant to get into the pool. "I'd rather lie poolside and work on my tan," he'd say. Or, "Tim, I love you man, but frolicking around in the pool, bare chest to bare chest, will bring our friendship to a new, slightly disturbing, level."

"Shut up and trust me."

"Oh all right."

I entered the pool first while Denis lifted Mike from his chair and gently placed him in my arms. "Oy, this water is cold!" he exclaimed.

"*Oy?*" I teased.

"I don't take shrinkage lightly," he countered.

Denis and I took turns carrying Mike around in the pool. I threatened to dunk him a few times. He threatened to pee on me. So I refrained.

At each visit, after our venture into the pool, there was one more task: giving Mike a shower. The Joneses built a large, easily-accessible shower for Jeff. Denis and I wheeled Mike in and transferred him onto the bench. We were still in our swimsuits. One day, after lathering Mike in lavender-scented soap, I looked at him, then Denis, and burst into hysterical laughter. This was *not* the sort of threesome I'd ever fantasized for myself in a shower.

Denis looked confused, and mildly insulted, as if I were laughing at him. Mike's expression remained unchanged; he was accustomed to our unexplained fits of laughter. True to form, he teased: "Is this scent too *manly* for you?"

"No offense, guys, but I always envisioned a three-way shower much differently. Don't get me wrong, you're great shower partners, but I would much prefer Jessica Alba and Scarlett Johansson."

Mike and Denis started laughing like hyenas. "Sorry, Tim," said Denis, "just another shower with the Berkson boys!"

Chapter 5

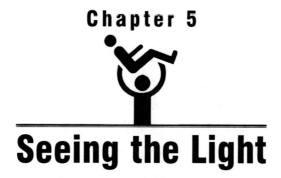

Seeing the Light

"Encouragement is the oxygen of the soul."
Anonymous.

I've made many an important life decision on the pot. The bathroom is a quiet place where I can shut out the world, gather my thoughts, and take care of business. This day was no different. It was late August. I was set to go back to school to get my master's degree in education. School and I never mixed well, and I wasn't looking forward to going back, but it seemed like the logical step.

After my morning run, I dialed my best friend, David. As the phone rang, I felt the call of nature and went to the bathroom to answer. David, on the other hand, did not answer.

As I placed the phone next to the sink, it rang. "Hello?" It was Denis.

"Hey Tim, how are you buddy?"

"Oh, hi, Denis! Great. Just sitting down – relaxing. What's up?"

"Wanted to touch base with you, see how you're doing. Are you ready for school?"

"Well I can't say I'm really ready for school, but it is what it is. How's the family?"

"Everyone's good. Except Mike. Cindy bought a house in Rockford and won't be returning as Mike's aide. Not to mention, all of Mike's teachers are new."

At Springman, a student stays on a team for two years with the same classmates and teachers to maintain continuity. Eighth grade meant the start of a new rotation. To make matters worse, Dan Walsh, head of student services and an important advocate of Mike's, had accepted a principal position in another district.

"Wow! Nobody's coming back? Not even his aide? That sucks! How's Mike doing?"

"He's taking it hard. You know Mike, he loves school. Now, he doesn't feel like going." He paused. "Wow, I never thought I'd ever say those words."

"Yeah – I bet."

"Well, Tim. Like you said, it is what it is."

My heart sank. "You know what, Denis? Fuck school! I'm working with Mike."

"You have to go to school, Tim." Denis worried that my decision was abrupt and reckless.

"Thing is, going back to school was something that sounded good to everyone else. I want to work with Mike."

"I don't know what to say. Thank you, Tim."

"You tell Mike that Batman and Robin have signed on for another season."

Working with Mike felt right to me. I hung up with Denis and flushed grad school away.

On Mike's first day, as I wheeled him to class, we overheard a couple of kids walking beside us discussing the Chicago Bears. Mike chimed in on their conversation, and one of them looked at me, utterly perplexed, and said, "He can speak?"

"Yeah," I replied angrily. "He can hear, too."

I restrained myself from clocking the kid. Mike simply shrugged it off. He had experienced that kind of ignorance for thirteen years, and such comments rarely bothered him. So often, Mike's peers were quick to judge and quick to say something inappropriate. Even certain of his teachers presumed Mike to be "slow," basing their presumption upon the wheelchair, not the person.

When we entered his next class, we were greeted by a gregarious social studies teacher, Mr. Steve Lesniak.

Mr. L. recognized Mike's heightened intellect almost immediately, and he embraced Mike with great enthusiasm. Mr. L. began the first class by asking students to share the first word they ever spoke.

I whispered to Mike, "My first word was *ball*."

"That doesn't surprise me," he retorted.

Later, a girl with a reputation for French kissing the boys said that her first word was "no." Mike laughed. "Yeah, right," he murmured. I broke into laughter, distracting the class.

On the way out, Mr. L. stopped Mike and me. "What was so funny?" he asked, his tone serious.

"Um…" I replied. Without hesitation, Mike shared his funny quip. To our surprise, Mr. L. laughed. "Good one," he said. "See you tomorrow."

Mike loved Mr. L.'s class. His assignments challenged Mike, and class discussions allowed him to exhibit his vocabulary and inventive logic. I enjoyed watching his peers' faces when he made a perceptive comment or posed an insightful question.

I wanted to tell the class how hard Mike worked. He worked with his family for countless hours on homework, relying on them to write answers and turn his textbook pages. What might take the average student an hour took Mike two or three hours to complete. Mike never complained. He thrived on learning.

One day, Mr. L. requested that Mike stay after class. "I've heard that before," Mike whispered.

"Don't worry," I said.

Mr. L. bent down on one knee, making eye contact with Mike.

"Are you proposing to me?" Mike asked.

Mr. L. laughed. "No," he replied. "I have an idea. I would like to make a thingamajig that when you press a button, a red light illuminates above your head. That way, you don't have to ask Tim to prop your arm when you want to raise your hand in class."

"That would be awesome!" Mike exclaimed, thrilled at the prospect of independence, even with something so seemingly minor.

Mr. L. (a.k.a. MacGyver) constructed the "thingamajig" from wire, a small boat light, and true grit. "Well, Mike," I said after Mr. L. attached the contraption to Mike's chair, "if you lose your electricity, you can still finish your homework under the light."

Chapter 6

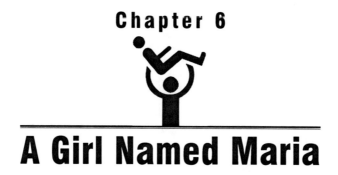

A Girl Named Maria

"I bet she smells like exotic fruit."
Mike Berkson

"The most beautiful sound I ever heard:
Maria, Maria, Maria..."

Y ou could almost hear every hormone-driven thirteen-year-old boy at Springman singing *Maria* from *West Side Story* while staring and drooling whenever the new girl walked by. Every boy except Mike; he only had eyes for Jenna, a sweet girl with a cute smile. He droned on about her for hours.

Jenna lived a couple of blocks from the Berksons and chilled with Mike and David now and then. She was the only girl who paid him any attention, and I determined that his crush resulted from lack of options. No offense to Jenna, but I decided to broaden his horizons.

During lunch break one Tuesday afternoon, I noticed Maria seated nearby. I whispered to Mike, "Pretty girl at 11 o'clock."

He looked confused. "Tim, it's 12:30."

I shook my head and laughed. "OK, little man. You want to learn something new?"

"What?"

"Picture yourself in the middle of a giant clock. At 11 o'clock, the hour hand points up and to the left. So, when a buddy tells you 'pretty girl at 11 o'clock' or any variation thereof, just look in the direction of the hour hand, and boom! Pretty girl appears!"

"Appears from where?"

"Listen dope, it's not magic. The pretty girl is there to begin with. The tactic is a subtle way for friends to point out pretty girls without physically pointing like a fool."

"Oh, why didn't you just say that in the first place?"

"Mike, we are wasting precious time here. Just look a little to your left."

When Mike laid eyes on her, his jaw dropped. He stopped breathing momentarily, mesmerized by this newly discovered treasure.

"She is beautiful," he said. "Like an angel."

"Easy there, pal. Don't get carried away."

From that moment on, Mike had three passions—school, movies and Maria.

When I was thirteen, I had a huge crush on a girl named Lauren. I stared. I drooled. I attempted to wave, once. But she never noticed me. I never approached her and simply said, "Hi." I was chicken.

Mike is no chicken. But we knew nothing about Maria. At that point, we didn't even know she *was* Maria. Later that day, Mike glanced at me contemplatively and whispered, "Tim, I'm in love. And I don't even know her name."

"We will find out about her," I assured him. "I'm on the case. In no time, you will be old friends. Maybe even lovers." I winked at my poor little love-struck friend.

After lunch, we followed ten steps behind her. She disappeared into a crowd of kids as she ascended the stairs. With that, we determined that she was an eighth grader on another student team. "First piece of the puzzle," I declared. Mike was not impressed.

"Wow. That was cool," he said sarcastically. "You really know what you're doing."

"What did you expect? To propose before Mr. L's class?"

"Well…no…but…"

"Mike, I've made and have yet to make more mistakes with girls than I care to mention. But with mistakes comes experience, and with experience, success. We will find out about her. I promise."

The next morning, we decided to take the scenic route to the library as classes upstairs were letting out. By a stroke of fate, or well-calculated timing, the girl whom Mike dubbed "the angel of Springman" exited a classroom and started walking in our direction. As soon as she appeared, Mike tensed.

"Relax buddy," I whispered. I hoped she might notice Mike and smile. Alas, someone shouted, "Hey Maria!" and she turned her back. I smiled at Mike and whispered, "The most beautiful sound…." Maria walked away, but we were content with this new, vital bit of information.

We took the same scenic route every day thereafter. Every time Mike caught a glimpse of Maria, he whispered sweet nothings into the wrong ear, mine: "She is an angel" and "I bet she smells like exotic fruit" and "My heart skips two beats whenever she walks by."

"When did you start writing romantic poetry?" I teased.

"Tim," he whimpered, "she tortures my soul."

"No worries, my smitten partner in crime. We will take many trips to the library."

When I greeted Mike the next morning, he had a twinkle in his eye and his signature sly smile. "Guess who I talked to at David's basketball game last night?"

"Um ... Quentin Tarantino?"

"No!"

"Jerry Seinfeld?"

"*Maria!* I talked to Maria!" I loved his exuberance. "She walked by and smiled. I smiled back. She sat next to me, and we talked!" He spoke quickly and with great excitement. "And guess what?!"

"What?"

"She *does* smell like exotic fruit!"

Our daily 10 a.m. trips to the upstairs hallway became a ritual. We timed them perfectly so that just as Mike exited the elevator, Maria walked by. Sometimes she waved and said "hello." Sometimes, to Mike's immeasurable pleasure, she stopped and engaged in small talk.

One day, Mike and I were a little late. We got to the elevator just as classes let out. Fearing we might miss her, Mike demanded that we floor it once the elevator doors opened.

"Tim, hurry! We can make it!" I obliged. We sped down the ramp outside the elevator and lost control. Boom! We hit the railing, and

Mike's arm got stuck between the wheelchair and rail. His arm hurt, but missing Maria hurt more.

I wheeled Mike to the nurse's office. Upon entering the waiting room, Mike gasped. "Maria," he uttered involuntarily.

She looked over. "Hi, Mike. What are you doing here?"

"Oh, Tim just ran me into a railing."

Maria turned to me. "That wasn't very nice."

"I didn't mean to," I replied, biting my tongue so as not to blame her for the injury.

"You'd better be more careful with Mike," she scolded. "I don't want to see him hurt." With that, she left, waving goodbye to Mike and shooting me a watchful glance.

"It was meant to be," Mike crooned.

With Christmas quickly approaching, I devised a brilliant plan. "Mike, what would you say if I got Maria to kiss you?"

"How?"

I attached mistletoe to Mike's chair.

"Um … OK," Mike said. "Make me look stupid. That'll work."

"Just trust me."

We made our way to the cafeteria. Mike felt uneasy. "Trust me," I repeated.

Maria, and her friends Kristen and Kat, approached him. "Mistletoe!" I exclaimed. "You get to kiss Mike."

Without hesitation, one by one, the girls kissed Mike—Kristen first, then Kat. (Mike later told me that Kat licked his forehead. "They don't call her Kat for nothing," he joked.)

And ... finally ... Maria leaned over and kissed Mike on the lips. The girls giggled and rushed off to class, leaving Mike in a daze.

"Wow," he sighed.

Was it a dream? *I've just kissed a girl ... named Maria. And suddenly I've found ... how wonderful a sound ... can be!*

Chapter 7

Welcome to the Family

"Life is either a daring adventure or nothing."
Helen Keller

The forthcoming eighth grade trip to Washington, D.C., begged the inevitable question: "Do you think Maria will be there?"

"Well," I said, glancing at the clock. "It's about that time. Let's mosey on upstairs." We had something besides the usual gawking to do.

"Now, Mike," I directed as we rode the elevator, "just say, 'Hey, Maria. What's up? Are you going on the D.C. trip?' Keep it simple, OK?"

"Got it."

However often Mike spoke with Maria, he never got control of his nerves. Upon the sight of her, his body tensed and filled with butterflies. He compensated for this uneasiness by spouting out four- and five-syllable words that, to the typical tween, resembled a foreign language and, without fail, met with a baffled stare and a single-sylla-ble, "Huh?"

Like clockwork, Maria appeared the moment the elevator doors opened.

"Hi, Mike!"

"Um ... hey ... hi." Mike cleared his throat. "Hi-hi Maria."

She smiled. "Hi."

"What ... is ... up?" Mike said, mechanically and with great effort.

Uh oh, I thought.

"Not much," she replied with a smile, wholly aware of her affect on Mike and enjoying every moment – not in a mean way, but in an appreciative way.

"I was just ... um ... wondering if you are going on the trip. On the-the D.C. trip?" He struggled not to meander into complex vocabu-lary, and I regretted giving him advice. He might have spoken another language, but at least he wouldn't have sounded constipated.

"You bet! Are you?"

"Yes," Mike replied.

"Well, I have to get to class. Bye, Mike!"

"Bye..."

As she walked away, Mike finally took a breath. "Wow," he sighed.

"Good job," I said, patting his head.

"Don't patronize me," he retorted. "If I could, I'd slap myself in the face right now."

"I'm willing to oblige," I teased.

"You know," Mike said, with a devilish grin. "I heard there's a pool. Maybe I will see Maria in a bikini."

"Easy there, fella! How will I explain the sudden heart attack to your parents?"

"At least you can tell them I went with a smile," he replied. "Hmmmm … I wonder what color it is…"

Traveling with Mike had its advantages: We skipped the long lines at security and got to the gate with enough time to grab a bite. As the gate agent prepared for boarding, a flight attendant arrived with an "aisle chair." The narrow contraption ,with a tall, straight back designed to wheel Mike up and down the aisle if necessary, resembled a torture device.

"People will call me Hannibal Lector!"

"I bet it's more comfortable than it looks," I said, unconvincingly.

Mike and I boarded first, and as each of his peers walked by, Mike lowered his voice and said, "Hello, Clarise." A few kids laughed, while the others most likely had been banned from R-rated movies. *Amateurs,* I thought. When I noticed Maria boarding, I nudged Mike, and he prepared to give his best rendition of Mr. Hopkins.

"Hello, Clarise."

Maria look at him, confused. "Um … it's Maria." Mike's shoulders slumped.

"Don't sweat it, pal!" I said. "You'll get your chance to impress Miss Maria."

"Shhhh," he pleaded. "She'll hear you."

"Mike, she's fifteen rows back. I doubt she has superhuman ears."

"Never *ass*ume," Mike chided. He sighed. "Her ears are cute, aren't they?" I rolled my eyes and settled in for the three-hour flight.

While his peers gossiped, laughed, and threw plastic cups at one another behind him, Mike looked ever so uncomfortable, strapped in every which way by five seatbelts. True to form, Mike cracked jokes the entire ride.

"Off to see Archie Bunker's chair!" he exclaimed.

With arms flailing and head shaking, I channeled Edith: "Oh, Archie…"

"Will you shut up, huh?!" Mike countered.

We were greeted in D.C. by bitter Chicago cold and Lake Michigan winds. "I guess the weather took first class," Mike said, teeth chattering while we waited for the bus.

"Great! Just great!" I shouted when the bus, sans handicap lift, arrived. I looked at Jason, the aide to another disabled student and my back-up assistant to Mike, and said, "Well my friend, this weekend just got a lot more challenging." After everyone boarded the bus, I carried Mike to his seat, strapped him in, and then loaded his chair.

Cold and fatigued, I looked at Mike and said, "That wasn't in the brochure."

"Just another day in the lives of Mike and Tim," he replied. "What did you expect?"

I laughed. "True."

We made it to the hotel by 9 p.m., and our rumbling bellies rejoiced at the sight, and scent, of hot pizza awaiting our arrival. Jason, Andy, Mike and I shared a room. Andy, Jason's student, was mobile but developmentally challenged, having an aptitude of a fourth or fifth grader. I tuned to ESPN, anxious to watch Yao Ming's debut against

64

Shaq as the Rockets took on the Lakers. Yao Ming blocked three of Shaq's shots in the first quarter. "That's it, Yao!" Jason shouted. "Don't let Shaq in your kitchen!"

"Yeah! Hit him with a spatula!" Andy exclaimed, delighting in this "guy's night" camaraderie that he was not accustomed to.

"Jab him with a fork!" I yelled.

"Lacerate him with a ladle!" shouted Mike.

"Pummel him with a frying pan!" Jason bellowed.

"Mash his potatoes!" Andy roared, grinning from ear to ear. With that, we fell into fits of laughter for hours.

As the night came to a close, I gave Mike his medication, brushed his teeth, changed him into pajamas, and lay him on his mat that consisted of a few quilts on the floor. Mike did not want to share a bed with me. "Why not?" I teased. "Do I stink?"

"No, you snore. Loudly."

In truth, he feared falling off the bed or me kicking him off the bed (not deliberately, of course).

The alarm sounded promptly at 6:15 a.m. I longed to press the snooze button, but the thought of jeopardizing Mike's day jolted me awake. Mike was already awake, ever the bad sleeper.

I got Mike to the bathroom and commenced with the daily routine—give meds, brush teeth, pajamas off, diaper change, clothes on. Since Andy required less maintenance, Jason helped me with the production. I glanced at the time. It was 7:13 a.m.

"Son of a bitch! We're late!" I exclaimed, and quickly caught myself. While Mike is accustomed to my occasional curse-word ridden outbursts, Andy is not. "Oops," I said to Jason.

"No worries," he said.

On the way to breakfast, I pictured Andy, with those big, puppy dog eyes, looking at his mother and innocently asking, "Mom, what's a son of a bitch?"

Breakfast consisted of cereal and toast, for the reserved – and, for the brave, eggs and hash browns. After breakfast, the trip director, Mr. Buzard, gave Jason and me walkie-talkies in case I needed to call on him for assistance. We met the bus outside the hotel and were greeted by our animated bus driver/tour guide, James.

Then I proceeded with what became known as the "transfer." I lifted Mike out of his chair, James loaded his chair into the luggage compartment, and Jason and I carried Mike onto the bus, careful not to sacrifice any of his limbs in the process. Once seated, I strapped him in with five seatbelts, similar to how he'd been strapped into the instrument of torture. The "transfer" and "transfer in reverse" would occur at every stop.

After just glancing over the day's itinerary, my back hurt. Today's docket included Mount Vernon, Old Town Alexandria, Grant Memorial, Pentagon City Mall, National Cathedral, National Zoo, National Geographic Explorers Hall, Lincoln Memorial, and finally, the Vietnam and Korean War Memorials.

We arrived at Mount Vernon shortly after sunrise, executed the transfer, and took in the beautiful landscape, brimming with historic significance. We spent ninety minutes at the estate and gift shop, executed transfer in reverse, and proceeded to Old Town, Alexandria. Along the way, James kept the busload of tweens entertained, remarking on significant sights, regaling us with factoids, and asking trivia questions.

After taking in the sights and sounds of Old Town, again with transfer and transfer in reverse, we arrived at the National Zoo. Mike and I had little interest in watching pandas frolic about while reciting the customary "ooohs" and "ahhhs." We were on a mission – to find a bathroom with a changing table suitable for Mike.

Whenever we visit a public place, be it a restaurant or a zoo, locating suitable facilities for Mike often proves difficult or impossible. "Improvise," Denis told me when I expressed my concerns to him. "Or pray to the Almighty Toiletor, God of the Lavatory."

But the bathroom gods were not with us on this cold January morning. After an exhaustive search, we did come upon a bathroom with a sturdy, long counter and a sink, not the ideal but adequate. Determined to change Mike quickly, I forgot to position Jason as a lookout man. As I placed Mike on the counter, a man and his young son walked in. They froze at the sight of a tall teenager strewn over the counter, legs dangling in the sink basin. A look of disgust washed over the father's face, a look of curiosity over his son's. I looked at him, smiled, and went about my business. He grabbed the boy's hand and rushed out of the room.

"What?!" I shouted after them. "Never see a man change another man's diaper before?!"

Mike laughed. "Yeah," he said. "I didn't want to go all medieval on his ass." For every awkward situation, Mike had the perfect movie quote.

We took a gander at the pandas, performed the transfer, and proceeded to the Pentagon City Mall for lunch and a little shopping.

Mike loves the mall. It is his sanctuary. "You shop more than a teenage girl with her daddy's credit card!" I told him. Every time we went to the mall, Mike walked out with a purchase. On that day he wanted *Stankonia* by OutKast. Purchase in hand, we continued to window shop. Mike noticed something. "Look!" he shouted. "It's a Maryland Terrapins hat. We've got to get that for James!"

On our way out, I noticed a little kid, maybe three years old, across the atrium staring at Mike as he walked past us in the opposite direction. He could not take his eyes off of him. Perhaps he thought Mike was a robot, or that the wheelchair was some cool new toy to add to his next Christmas list. I saw it coming but could do nothing to stop it: The poor little guy, eyes still on Mike, walked straight into a large planter, fell back, and his butt hit the floor with a thump. He sat up in a daze, and after the pause that's so typical as a child contemplates whether to cry, he burst into tears. His father, who had been walking a few steps ahead, rushed to his side. I couldn't help but laugh. Thus far, it was the most entertaining site in D.C.

"Come in, Agent Jason."

"Jason here. Line secure."

"Lunch digested. Transactions complete. Transfer executed flawlessly. Proceed to Lincoln Memorial and Supreme Court."

"Roger, that. Over and out."

"Hey, kids." Buzard's stern voice interrupted our parody. "These walkie-talkies aren't toys."

"Sorry sir," I said, barely able to contain my laughter.

"You're a regular Red Buttons," Mike said.

At the Lincoln Memorial, Mike and I rested atop the steps, amid the thirty-six Doric columns and under the inscriptions of the Gettysburg Address. This was where Martin Luther King, Jr. had delivered his renowned speech.

"I have a dream," Mike whispered.

"What's that, pal?"

"I have a dream that I will be judged by the content of my character, not by my wheelchair. I have a dream that able-bodied Americans will refrain from parking in handicap spaces. I have a dream that when a wheelchair-bound man strives for the cereal box on the top shelf, others do not walk by pretending not to notice."

I felt a tear wet my cheek. Mike looked at me and said, "I have a dream that I will see Maria in a bikini at the community center tomorrow." And the tears, as usual, turned to laughter.

"I can't guarantee the bikini," I said, "but we'll make your other dreams a reality someday. I promise."

Every landmark we visited was wheelchair friendly until we reached the Supreme Court. Unable to follow the others up the stairs, Mike and I were directed to another entrance. As we circled the entire building, guards stopped us now and then but continued to send us the wrong way. We found ourselves back at the base of the main stairs, where another security guard approached us.

"Can I help you?" he asked. He seemed condescending and accusing.

"Yes," Mike replied, insulted. He became sarcastic: "Isn't it obvious? We're going to ram my wheelchair into the building."

The guard's face flushed with anger, and I attempted to appease him with a smile. "It's been a long day," I said. "We're just looking for the nearest handicap entrance." He pointed in the direction from which we had come.

We turned around and circled the building again, only to find the entrance at the base of the steps, five feet from the guard.

Catching up with the class, we found the building rather anti-climactic. There wasn't much to see, as most areas were blocked off for construction. We returned to the bus, and after the transfer, Mike looked at me with a big smile. "I wonder if my name will be on the terrorist watch list now."

We arrived at the National Cathedral as the sun began to set and yawns permeated the busload. Mike asked to stay on the bus.

"I'm not the religious type," he said. I did not argue. I often wondered if Mike was angry with God, or any higher power, for his condition. I never asked.

After dinner, the class went to a play at the Kennedy Center. Mike felt tired, so we returned to the hotel. Jason and Andy joined us. Back at the room, we watched the Wizards game featuring number 23 —Michael Jordan.

Andy poked my shoulder. "Tim, can we build a tent for me to sleep in?"

"Sure," I replied. Andy smiled ear to ear. Jason and I used pillows and comforters to construct a semi-stable fort.

"I can't wait to sleep tonight!" Andy exclaimed.

Jason and I derived such pleasure from making our kids happy, and although we expected the fort to crash in the middle of the night, we felt a sense of pride in our accomplishment. Truly, the simple things in life, even if fashioned from sheets and pillows, are what make you happy.

I set the alarm for 6 a.m. with the expectation of another transfer-yet-fun-filled day—White House, Holocaust Museum, Ford's Theater, FDR Memorial, and the highly anticipated, potentially bikini-clad

Maria sighting at the community center. The forecast called for rain, and I prayed that Mother Nature might cut us a break.

The day began with a trip to the White House. We watched as the bus passed hundreds of antiwar protesters. While viewing the exterior of the White House, I bent over Mike to apply lotion to his dry hands. A security guard approached and requested that I forfeit the lotion. I conceded, bewildered. I offered him my umbrella as well. He shooed the umbrella away. "Those are permitted," he said and moved to the next student.

"Does it rain inside the White House?" Mike asked sarcastically.

"Maybe," I whispered. "To wash away all the bullshit."

Mike let out a loud chuckle, catching the attention of a few guards. "I hope he doesn't confiscate my laughter, too," Mike whispered.

At Ford's Theater, Mike and I were unable to join the group because the building was not handicapped accessible. We stayed on the bus, without complaint. On a small TV that James kept on the bus, we watched the Eagles play the Buccaneers for the NFC championship. I rooted for Tampa Bay, despite the odds against them, and much to my surprise, they were winning. I know Donovan McNabb is from Chicago, but I love to see the underdog win.

Later that day, as I steered Mike through the Holocaust Museum, chills permeated my body. We were reminded of the world's cruelty and darkness, alongside representations of courage, bravery and perseverance. At the Wall of Remembrance, you can light a candle and pray – for the victims, for the survivors, or for a world without war.

Although Mike is not religious and never prays, he asked that I light a candle on his behalf, having been moved by the exhibits. I tried to light one, to no avail, then tried another and continued to struggle. It was like a trick candle on a birthday cake.

"I can't get this damn candle to light," I murmured in frustration, forgetting my place. I hadn't spoken loudly, but my voice did carry, and Mike roared with laughter – and when the surroundings are inappropriate, laughter becomes even more contagious. I grabbed Mike's chair and wheeled him out of the room quickly while struggling to stifle my own laughter. Inevitably, I lost it. I tried to disguise my guffaws as sobs, wiping away pretend tears. I think it worked.

Our final stop was the FDR Memorial, which I couldn't wait to explore with Mike. "FDR spent his presidency in a wheelchair," I told Mike as the bus approached the memorial.

"Wow," Mike replied. "That's cool."

The tour guide expanded on the subject. "In August 1921, Roosevelt contracted an illness which resulted in his permanent paralysis from the waist down. For the rest of his life, Roosevelt refused to accept that he was permanently paralyzed, and he attempted a broad range of therapies. After he became president, he founded the National Foundation for Infantile Paralysis, now known as the March of Dimes."

"Cripples represent!" Mike shouted. His classmates roared and clapped.

After about fifteen transfers and countless miles walked, I felt tired and achy as we sat down to dinner.

"Time for the community center!" Mike exclaimed after we finished our meal. I didn't mind walking five more blocks, for the sake of my love-struck friend, but I first wanted to ensure that Maria would, in fact, be there. I left Mike with Jason and scoured the restaurant for Maria. I noticed her chatting with friends, so I moseyed over to eavesdrop.

"You girls have fun at the pool. I'm going back to the hotel to see *The Hot Chick* on HBO," Maria said. I rejoiced and rushed back to Mike to deliver the "disappointing" news. I omitted *The Hot Chick* detail, fearing that Maria's taste in movies would ruin Mike's fascination with her.

When Mike awoke the next morning, the final day of our trip, he proclaimed, "Today we see Archie Bunker's chair!"

"Will you shut up, huh?!" I yelled, still half asleep.

We packed our luggage and boarded the bus. Before our flight, there were two final stops – Arlington National Cemetery and the Smithsonian. On arriving at the Smithsonian, Mike and I were presented with yet another bathroom challenge, and we fruitlessly evoked the power of the gods. We found the customer service desk and asked directions to the handicap rest rooms.

"The bathroom stalls are equipped with bars for disabled individuals," she told us.

"We don't want a stall," I replied. "I need a changing table."

I looked at my watch. We had about thirty minutes to change Mike, see the chair, and return to the bus parked ten minutes away.

"Look," I continued. "I don't care if it's the boiler room or an administrative office, but I need a place to help my friend change into a new pair of under … undershorts."

"Well, the only changing table I know of is in the women's restroom."

I looked at Mike. "What do you say?"

He shrugged. "If we have to."

I checked the time—down to twenty-five minutes. Desperate times call for desperate measures. As I approached the door to the ladies room, a security guard stopped us.

"Excuse me," I said. "I have to use the changing table."

She got between us and the door. I opened my mouth, prepared to argue, when she halted my forthcoming tirade with her hand and said, "There's a private bathroom with a changing table down that hallway and to the left."

"Thank you!" I shouted as I ran with Mike down the hallway. Miraculously, the bathroom gods answered our call.

I changed Mike faster than ever before, returned him to his chair, and hurried out of the bathroom. We were down to twelve minutes. We rushed through the crowds at the National Museum of American History. We whizzed past Dorothy's ruby slippers from *The Wizard of Oz*. Almost there. We flew past Fonzi's leather jacket, *aieeeeeee!* We turned a corner, and *voila!* Archie Bunker's chair.

We neared the glass. "That's it, huh?" Mike said.

"Basically," I replied. "Pretty muuuch … just a chair."

The endeavor proved anticlimactic, but it was a symbol for us. In seeing it, we had accomplished something. Sometimes we set goals in life, and when we reach them, we say, "Is that all there is?" And sometimes, yeah, that's all there is. Yet there's always fun to be had in the journey.

After our final transfer, and transfer in reverse, Mike presented James with his token of appreciation, the Maryland Terrapins hat. He loved it. We boarded the plane. This time Mike refrained from his Hanibal Lector impersonation. We were all tired.

The Berksons greeted us outside the airport, and we regaled them with stories – from lacerating ladles to Archie Bunker's chair. When we arrived at my place, I looked at Mike and said, "School tomorrow?"

"No way!" he replied.

"Thank God!" I exclaimed. "I'm sleeping in."

Denis walked me to the door and put his arm around me. "Tim, Mike couldn't have experienced this without you. Our family will always be indebted to you. You are our angel."

"What I did this weekend was no big deal," I told him. "That's what families do for each other."

Denis hugged me and looked me in the eye. "Welcome to the family," he said.

Chapter 8

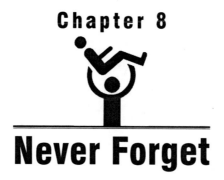

Never Forget

*"To be good is noble, but to show others how
to be good is nobler and no trouble."*
Mark Twain

Mike's final social studies project required him to direct and produce "The Team Quest Video." The short film summed up what the students learned that year and involved interviewing his peers and recreating certain projects to demonstrate how the students had worked as a team.

Mr. L. assigned a couple students to assist, and Mike channeled his inner Tarantino. He transformed a rather boring topic into a collage of creative angles, with sharp editing and a comedic edge. Mike enjoyed every moment as he fell completely into his element. The class loved it.

"We'll see you on the red carpet some day," Mr. L. proclaimed. "Remember the name, kids – Mike Berkson. The man. The myth. The legend!"

Alas, someone did forget Mike's name. At the class party, students were given T-shirts with classmates' names listed on the back. I grabbed one of the shirts from the box and searched for Mike's name.

"You've got to be shitting me!" I exclaimed.

"What?" Mike asked.

"Sorry, pal. Your name isn't on the shirt."

Mike let out a sigh. "Erased from existence. I suppose this was all a dream." He attempted to mask his disappointment with sarcasm. But he was hurt.

"Mikey, I have an idea – if you don't mind defacing the shirt."

"Deface away, my friend. Deface away." I found a black marker and proceeded to write on the back of the shirt.

"What are you writing?"

"You'll see," I teased.

"Tell me!" Mike pleaded.

I crossed the final T and revealed my magnum opus. For the rest of the day, Mike wore the shirt, marked by the words "NEVER FORGET."

When Mike told his dad about the mistake, Denis called the principal and left a passionate message, not exactly politically correct, demanding that the district reprint and redistribute all the shirts. The principal called the next day, apologized profusely, and said, "Regrettably, we cannot reprint the shirts for budget reason, but we will print a shirt for Mike that includes his name." Not good enough, we all thought.

"Tim?"

"Yeah, buddy?" I was helping Mike get ready for graduation as we reminisced about the year.

"Will you push me across the stage?"

"Really? Are you sure?" His question caught me by surprise. I expected that Denis or David would be walking with him.

"I'm sure."

"Of course I will! Thank you." I felt extraordinarily honored.

That night, when Mike's name was called, I pushed him across the stage. The crowd gave Mike a standing ovation. I slowed, allowing Mike to relish the moment. As we rejoined his class, I whispered, "How does it feel, Mike? You are the man! No one forgot you tonight."

He smiled and said, "Bye bye Springman," a reference to the play Bye Bye Birdie.

As we prepared to leave the stage at the end of the ceremony, I asked Mike if he wanted Mr. L. to walk with us. "Yes!" he exclaimed. I motioned for Mr. L. to join us, and we proceeded to exit amid another standing ovation.

As we walked off the stage, I turned to Mr. L. and mouthed the words, "Thank you." A tear fell down his cheek. Later that night, Mr. L. wrote this in Mike's yearbook: "Mike, you have inspired me to pursue things greater than I thought possible. I wish you all the happiness you brought into my life, times ten."

Mike is still waiting for the shirt with his name on it.

Chapter 9

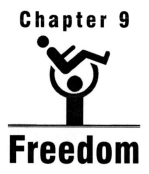

Freedom

"It does not matter how slowly you go so long as you do not stop."
Confucius

I could not believe the size of Mike's high school, Glenbrook South. The expansive campus could be intimidating to any freshman, especially from the viewpoint of a wheelchair. Most of the 2,500 students navigating the hallways found their way around with ease. Mike and I felt lost. Pushing his wheelchair through a sea of teens proved daunting.

I sensed Mike's customary high spirits deteriorating. I think reality struck him hard. He was getting older, knew he would require an aide for the remainder of his adult life, and was watching the world rush by – without him. He witnessed his identical twin enjoying sports and laughing with friends. Those friends were without a care in the world, taking for granted the things he would never be able to take for granted.

On his third day, while we waited for the elevator, three older students approached us. "Can we ride in the elevator with you?" asked the tallest of the three.

"Why?" Mike inquired.

"Elevators are cool," he replied. "And we don't want to take the stairs."

"Be thankful you can take the stairs," Mike told them. "I wish I could." They walked away.

During our bathroom break that day, I noticed sadness splashed across Mike's face. "Tim," he said. "Sometimes my smile is fake, and I'm getting tired of faking it." I stood there, shocked. "I know, I'm damned good. Aren't I?" he said sarcastically. His toned changed, darkened. "I'm so angry. I'm angry at all the people who can walk. They are so passive. They don't notice any of the world around them. They move so quickly to their next stage of existence. And here I sit in one spot for what seems like an eternity, and they keep on going in their own direction, taking everything I would cherish for granted."

"How can I help you?"

"No one can help me. I'm stuck. I hate this place. I hate these people. Nobody listens to me. People ignore me. Everybody looks at me like I'm some freak. I'm not – I'm just like they are! Everyone thinks they know what's best for me. They don't! They're not stuck in this chair – they're not in my head – they have no idea what it's like, and everyone's so fixed on 'making my quality of life better' that nobody thinks to ask me what I want. I'm sick of it. I'm so sick of it!" Mike was unraveling before me.

There was a knock on the door. "We need to get out of here, little man."

"I'll be all right, Tim."

"I know, Mike. I know." We left our emotions in the bathroom that morning, only to find them waiting there for us the next day. After I changed him, he uttered words that I will never forget.

"Tim, I just want to end it. I want to take my life. And you know what the sad thing is? I want to kill myself because I cannot do anything, but if I had the ability to kill myself, I would not want to."

We stared at each other, crying. Then, suddenly, we started to laugh. Maybe laughter was our way of coping with Mike's reality.

"Mike, I want to share something with you. Nine years ago, I fell into a deep depression."

"You were depressed?"

"You think we able-bodied folk are immune to depression? Depression doesn't discriminate," I said.

"Wow."

"It began with a crash diet—I cut out all fat. I lost weight, and to some degree I lost my mind. Turns out, your brain needs fat to function properly. I became hyper. I couldn't sleep, overcome by unending, racing thoughts about … I don't even remember. After one week without sleep, I went to a doctor. He labeled me a manic depressive. I questioned his diagnosis, never having been depressed a day in my life. 'You have the classic symptoms,' he told me, and wrote me a prescription for medication.

"That was May. By September, I had been on a series of medications, and I went from manic to despondent. I did not feel like myself with these various medications coursing through my veins. I felt lost and confused. The meds made me feel powerless and unmotivated. I dropped out of school. I dropped out of life." Mike looked at me with concern.

"Mike, it gets worse. I felt like you. I wanted to end my life. I cried myself to sleep nightly. I even devised a plan – go to the Edgebrook train station with my pillow and Walkman, and lay on the train tracks until I fell asleep forever." Tears were streaming down my face, soaking my shirt.

"What stopped you?"

"I asked myself a question. How would my parents deal with it? I thought about the effect it would have on the people I love – the people that love me. That scared me straight." I hid my face behind my hands, sobbing.

"I'm sorry, Tim." I felt Mike wanting to place his hand on my shoulder. "Don't get your shirt too wet with tears," he said. "People will think I peed on you again."

I laughed and dried my eyes. "That November, I went to my doctor and told him I wanted off the medications. 'You will be in a mental institution within six months,' he told me. I looked him in the eye and said with conviction, 'You're wrong.' He looked at me like I was crazy, but it was the most sane I had felt in months. I weaned myself off the medication and began to feel like myself again."

"And now here you are," Mike said. "You're not in a mental institution. You're in a bathroom changing a teenager's diaper."

I smiled. "I wouldn't have it any other way. You know, I often wonder what would have happened if I'd never asked myself that question about what would happen to the people I love."

"And, what do you come up with?"

"I don't hold onto the thought long enough to formulate a scenario. Not important now. What is important now is you. Mike, we were brought into each other's lives for a reason, even if that reason is not apparent now. My life is far better with you and your family in it."

A single tear fell down Mike's cheek. "Tim, I feel the same way. You are so much fun. No one believes me when I mention you are twenty-nine."

I laughed wholeheartedly, causing a little debris to shoot from my nose and hit Mike's arm. "Sorry about that, Mike," I said, wiping his arm. "That little guy couldn't wait to escape. Now he is free."

"Tim, so are we."

Nine years earlier, I'd decided to have fun with my life. Every day above ground was a great day. I couldn't control the weather or the remarks of ignorant kids, but I could control my attitude.

As Mike and I went through the rest of the day, we felt changed and better armed to tackle the crowded hallways. When I said goodbye to Mike that day, I leaned over and whispered, "There's no crying in high school." He smiled. From then on, we focused on laughter.

Chapter 10

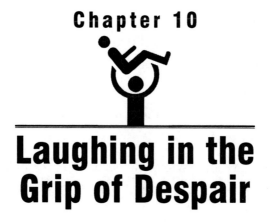

Laughing in the Grip of Despair

"We all have our wheelchairs."
Denis Berkson

Announcer: Listen to what some of the most acclaimed broadcasting personalities are saying about *The Mike Berkson Show*.

Howard Cosell: This is Howard Cosell. I have never heard such an invigorating show in all the years I've been dead. Marv, what do you think?

Marv Albert: Yes!

Walter Cronkite: I am Walter Cronkite. *The Mike Berkson Show* is top dawg. That's the way it is. Dennis Miller, what do you have to say?

Dennis Miller: Listen, Cha-Cha. *The Mike Berkson Show* makes Stephen Hawking look like a community theater performance of *Les Miserables* in Baghdad.

Announcer: So remember, listen to *The Mike Berkson Show* every Saturday at 10 a.m. on WGBK 88.5, Glenbrook South's student station. Holla!

By the second semester of ninth grade, Mike settled in and began to thoroughly enjoy school, especially his broadcasting class with Mrs. Del Kennedy. When she played Mike's latest masterpiece, his self-made radio show commercial, the class applauded in appreciation of his keen humor. I enjoyed watching him soak up the praise. I soaked up a little, too: I was the voice talent.

I usually tuned in to Mike's show. He sounded fluid and relaxed. One Saturday morning, I decided to call and chime in on a commentary about Pete Rose.

"We have a caller. Ralph from Chicago, you're on the air."

I tried to disguise my voice, and my laughter. "First of all, guys, great show, great show. I'm a little older than all of you, and I had the privilege of seeing Pete Rose play, live and on TV. As a baseball player, considering what he accomplished between the lines, there is no doubt he belongs in the Hall of Fame. Unfortunately, Mr. Rose committed the cardinal sin in baseball—wagering on the game."

One of Mike's cohorts replied, "Well, it is certainly great to get a call from an oldie. All we have is video and our parents' accounts. Have you any more to add?"

I heard Mike laughing in the background. He lost his radio composure. *Come on Mikey, you're better than that,* I thought.

"Yes. Although Rose finally admitted to betting on baseball, he does not deserve Hall of Fame status. What message will it send to all of the innocent little baseball fans out there? I hope Bud Selig does not reinstate him! Mr. Rose made his bed and must now sleep in its slimy, shame-ridden sheets."

Mike, now poised and self-assured, said, "Thanks for the call, Tim. You contributed a nice nugget of information to our commentary. See you Monday."

Another class that Mike adored was Honors English, except for one book – *Jane Eyre*. I agreed. After reading three pages to him, I stopped.

"Sorry, dude. I can't. I don't know what I'm reading. I can't take it!"

His teacher, Mrs. Debbie Middleton, knew Mike well. She exploited his strengths. Having noticed his distaste for *Jane Eyre*, she decided to give him an unconventional assignment. "Mike, do you have access to a video camera?"

Sure do," he answered.

"Well, Mr. Berkson, I want you to record your thoughts on *Jane Eyre*. Any way you want to. Film it, and I'll play it."

"Any way I want?" Mike asked, awaiting the inevitable attached strings.

"Any way. Mike, if you hate it, explain why."

The wheels inside his innovative mind were spinning furiously.

One week later, Mike entered the classroom, masterpiece in hand. "I'm ready, Mrs. Middleton."

The short film displayed the book lying flat on the floor. Mike's voice sounded in the background. "This is how I felt about the book." He proceeded to roll his chair over the book until the pages were strewn across the room. The camera cut to Mike as he spun off into a rap.

"…There she goes, down the aisle towards wedded bliss. Oh, what's that? Another depressing twist. Jane's future hubby has himself a crazy wifey. Poor lil' Jane … Charlotte, why'd you have to make it so boring? Your long-winded prose left me snoring. The plot needs slapstick and laughter, a lil' action, a happier ever after."

The class exploded into applause.

Meanwhile, Mike was swept up in a happily-ever-after story of his own. Maria and her exotic scent were a faint memory, and Mike had a new love interest – Hannah. Hannah walked short distances with help but otherwise used a wheelchair. She could not talk and communicated via a talking computer. She was never without a smile.

"She asked me out," Mike told David and me excitedly.

"I figured that," I replied. He looked at me inquisitively. "Mike, you're not the type to make the first move."

"You know me too well, man."

"Mike and Hannah sitting in a tree…," David teased.

"Yeah, I'd like to see you hoist me into a tree."

"Don't tempt me."

"So … don't keep me in suspense! I want details," I prodded.

"She came over a couple weeks ago. We watched *Meet the Parents*, then went to the theater to see *Meet the Fockers*." Mike loved telling the story.

"Mikey, you animal! My boy's all growns up and he's all growns up," I said, wiping away a fake tear. "Did you make a move?!"

"No," he replied sheepishly. "She did put her hand on mine during the movie."

"That Hannah is a sly fox!" I exclaimed. "When are you lovebirds going out again? I want to see Don Juan in action."

"Probably in a couple weeks."

"Great. If you ever need a chaperone, let me know."

In the ensuing weeks, Mike came down with a cold. Denis called me one lazy Saturday afternoon. "He is not doing well, Tim."

"Anything I can do?"

"Funny you should ask," Denis replied. "Linda's taking Mike to the doctor. Will you go with her?"

I didn't need to say "absolutely!" I merely asked, "When?"

When Mike comes down with the slightest of colds, his parents and doctor take great precautions to ensure that it does not develop into a more serious, and potentially life threatening, condition. What you and I might refer to as a "little cold" takes a big toll on Mike. He grapples with a persistent cough that keeps him up at night and inhibits his ability to breathe with ease. Not to mention, he cannot wipe the mucus and spit from his face, and amid his coughing must constantly request assistance.

After the doctor visit, his health improved. Medications were helping, and the Turnabout Dance was coming up.

Hannah asked Mike to be her date, and he desperately wanted to oblige. I volunteered as chaperone, as promised. On the evening of the dance, I felt even more excited than Mike.

A couple hours before the dance, Denis called. "Tim, Mike's not well." My heart sank. "He can't go to the dance."

"I'm sorry, Denis. How is Hannah?"

"I delivered the corsage to her and a cookie Mike got her, frosted with the words 'I'm sorry.' She smiled from ear to ear. She gave me Mike's boutonniere and a drawing from her little sister of Mike and Hannah dancing. Tore my heart out."

That night, I reminisced about high school dances past. I remembered standing against a wall, too shy to ask a girl to dance. What a little fool. I thought of how gracious Mike and Hannah were amid such disappointment, and I would have given anything at that moment to bring that drawing to life.

After missing a week of school, Mike returned, happy and healthy, and we fell back into our usual routine. Between classes, Mike and I chilled on the bench outside the cafeteria and talked, discussing his latest project, a Sopranos episode, or his latest love interest, Hannah. Without fail, the maintenance man, Chuck Haley, stopped by to say hello.

Chuck reminisced about his days as a professional wrestler. "Want to know what they called me?" he asked Mike.

"The Round Mound of Ultrasonic Sound?" Mike teased.

"*The Round Mound?* Are you calling me fat, you little … jokester! No, they called me … (he channeled a deep, thunderous voice) … the Minnesota Mauler!"

Then Chuck described his signature move. "I'd trap my opponent in 'the grip of despair.' It was all over for him, Mikey. Want me to demonstrate on Tim?"

"Um…," I interrupted. "Why don't you grab some unsuspecting punk in the hallway?" I cleared my throat. "After all, I don't want to hurt you, Chuck."

He called my bluff. "Chicken…" he said under his breath. Mike laughed.

"OK," I conceded. "Lay it on me."

Chuck positioned himself behind me and placed his arms on my shoulders. "You see, Mike, you get them here, then bring your left arm around the neck." I shot Mike one of those "you owe me" looks.

Reaching around the top of my head with his right arm, Chuck proceeded to lock me in the "grip of despair." I was choking. Mike was laughing. After two seconds, which felt like two hours, Chuck released me.

He enjoyed flaunting his moves and recounting those happy memories. At times, as Chuck finished a story, I thought I saw a twinge of sadness in his eyes. I thought, perhaps, he once dreamt of becoming a famous wrestler, and somewhere on the way to wrestle-mania super-stardom, he fell in love, started a family, and chose more practical, less precarious means of providing support. Maybe he still daydreams, not with regret for the life he chose, but longing for that rush of adrenaline, the roar of the crowd, and the taste of blood on his lips. And now, he felt that time had passed him by. In some ways, he found a kindred spirit in Mike, as did so many others.

As Denis once said, "We all have our wheelchairs. Mike's happens to be visible."

Mike has attracted amazing people and experiences into his life, and I felt honored to be along for the ride. Mike was Batman, I was Robin. Mike was MJ and I was Scottie. He was the show. He is the show. He will always be the show.

Chapter 11

When One Door Closes...

"In the moments of decision, destiny is shaped."
Tony Robbins

I n December of Mike's freshmen year, I had applied for a local 911 dispatch job. By March, having received no response, I had forgotten about it.

Then, one late March morning, I received a letter announcing a written exam for the job, followed by a job simulation exam and a one-on-one interview. A week later, I took the exam alongside thirty-nine other applicants, of which three would be hired. I had a one in thirteen chance; I felt confident. I was among eighteen applicants to pass the written exam, progressing to the job simulation exam, and bettering my odds to one in six. Two weeks later, my chances were one in three, as I joined five applicants in proceeding to the interview phase. As I waited in the empty office for my interview, I felt positive and energized.

And, in that moment, it hit me. Mike. If I were hired, the job would start in May, a month before the end of the school year. While I had kept Denis and Linda abreast of the application process, we decided not to tell Mike until after the interview. When Jim, a tall, brawny man with a serious countenance and firm handshake, entered the room, I focused on the task. I answered each question with poise and certainty, and I even got Jim smiling by the interview's end.

Although my hire was not yet official, I wanted to warn Mike and my school supervisors that I might leave before the end of the school year. I decided to break the news to Mike in the place where our bond had strengthened the most – the bathroom. I changed him, transferred him back to his chair, and sat on the toilet.

"Tim, please don't do anything vile. I can't run." I half-laughed, half-sobbed. Tears rolled down my face.

"What's wrong?" Mike asked. I drifted off into a reverie, one similar to those corny sequences in chick flicks where a slow-motion montage of sappy moments plays out to even sappier music. In my mind, the montage – spilled Taco Bell, projectile urine, trash compactors, threesome showers – played out to Barbra Streisand's *The Way We Were*.

"Tim ... Tim! Are you OK?" Mike pulled me out of my montage sequence and into the moment I dreaded. "Are you feeling all right?"

"Mike, before I met you, I felt lost. Then you rolled into my life, and gave me direction. You gave me the momentum to move forward. I'm so grateful to you."

"Are you breaking up with me?" Mike said sarcastically. I cried more.

"Mike, I've applied for a job as a 911 dispatcher, and I've made it to the final interview phase. If I get the job, I start in May. I hate to leave you before the end of the school year, but..."

Mike sat there, speechless. That was the first time I could remember that happening. After what seemed to be an hour, he broke his silence.

"You have to do what's best for you. I understand."

"And no, I'm not breaking up with you." I smiled. "You are my best friend, my partner in crime, my comrade, my wingman..."

"I get it." Mike grinned. "Like matter cannot be created or destroyed, our bond is strong and will merely change shape."

"I guess chemistry comes in handy once in a while."

"Whoever replaces you has some big shoes to fill – and I mean that literally and figuratively." We laughed and went on with the day with brave faces.

I called Denis that night to check on Mike. "He's a little upset," Denis said. "He feels conflicted. He wants the best for you but will miss you terribly."

I felt conflicted as well. I did not want to leave Mike, but my finances were strained. I needed more income. I couldn't sleep that night, burdened by unending thoughts. I wanted the salary that more than doubled my current one, but not the job itself. It was not a long-term position, merely a temporary financial fix.

A week later I received a letter from Jim stating that, although he found me impressive, the positions had been given to three applicants with prior dispatch experience. I felt extreme disappointment and, surprisingly, overwhelming relief. I would get to finish off the year with Mike, and I learned something – that although I loved working with

Mike, the time had come to move on to new adventures. I decided not to return as Mike's aide the following year. I wanted to become a professional speaker, and as long as I felt comfortable in my job, I would not pursue it. Not working with Mike would force me to try.

After telling my supervisors at Glenbrook South that I would not return in the fall, I felt a sense of power. I made a tough decision and followed through with it. I felt in control. Naturally, that feeling was laced with a little fear. I alleviated the fear in the way that Mike had taught me – I redirected my focus. Since I was twenty-one, I'd wanted to speak before audiences and change people's lives for the better. I focused on making it happen.

In July, I got my break. A former colleague and old friend, Chad Carden, called with a job opportunity. He and his business partner, Adam Carroll, were starting a venture called National Financial Educators that toured colleges delivering a seminar called *The Money Game*. The seminar outlined sound and practical tips for creating financial stability while still in college. Chad requested that I come on board as vice president of development and as a speaker. The position would allow me to hone my speaking, marketing and sales skills, as well as increase my income.

I called Mike to share the exciting news.

"As Notorious B.I.G. would say, mo money mo problems," Mike teased.

"Well, I've experienced mo money problems than I care to mention, so I'll risk it." We laughed and discussed the coming school year, Mike's latest date with Hannah, and the Sox.

Chicago summers, which last from late May to late September, are like no other. Lake Michigan is magnificent. The skyline is stunning by

WHEN ONE DOOR CLOSES…

day and breathtaking by night. The city brims with delightful activity by day, and Navy Pier fireworks illuminate the sky by night.

Then, the beautiful weather bypasses fall and gives way to brutal winters. The bitter cold, augmented by killer winds, rips through the warmest of coats, scarves, flannel socks, gloves and ear muffs.

Chicago does not have a spring season; it has a schizo season. From March until May, the weather is utterly unpredictable – sixty degrees one day, ten the next. So, when summer finally arrives, we Chicagoans rejoice after eight months of oppression and indulge in four months of pleasure. And, as winter again reveals its ugly, brutally cold face, we whine. A lot.

For three years, I had associated the dreaded walk down the end-of-summer plank with the beginning of the school year with Mike. As I worked long hours in September, and the days shortened and became cooler, I began to miss Mike. We spoke frequently; however, I missed the theatrical bathroom breaks, the inside jokes, and the potential for adventure every day. At the same time, I felt keyed up and optimistic about the opportunities that my new position offered.

One Saturday evening that September, David was lounging on the couch watching *America's Most Wanted*, while Mike sat in his chair flipping through the channels in his room. Denis and Linda were at the Joneses for dinner. The phone rang; David answered. "Hello?" Hearing only shallow breaths, he hung up the phone. "Stupid prank," he grumbled and hopped back on the couch. Then, David thought he heard a noise outside the living room window. He muted the television and listened. He heard the noise again. Amid the rustling of trees, he heard someone trying to open the living room window. He ran into Mike's room, breathless. "Mike, someone's trying to break in!"

"Yeah, right," Mike replied, assuming his brother was joking. Besides, what could he do? Run? Call for help?

"I'm serious!" David urged. "What should I do?"

"OK, calm down," Mike replied, still doubtful. "Call the neighbors."

The doorbell rang, and David nearly fainted. "Just get the door," Mike said.

"What?! No way! You get the door!"

"If I could…" He paused. "Push me to the door."

"But what if … what if…" David could not formulate a sentence.

"Just push me to the door." Mike wasn't afraid of anything. David conceded and pushed Mike to the front door. The bell rang again. David jumped.

"Who is it?" Mike said. No answer.

David's trembling hand extended to the knob and opened the door, slowly. I pressed my face between the door and the frame. "Here's Timmy!"

David came at me quick and sucker punched my stomach. "You jerk! You scared me half to death!"

Mike laughed hysterically. "That was awesome! Do it again."

David continued to punch me, and I wrestled him to the ground as his anger transformed into hilarity. The three of us laughed for an hour – David and me on the floor and Mike in his chair, in the Berksons' foyer, the door still open. Passersby probably thought we were crazy.

When we regained our composure, I compensated David for my practical joke with ice cream. While at the ice cream shop, Mike and

David filled me in on their first couple weeks of school – the classes they liked and the classes they hated, the pretty girls and the ugly teachers. Mike enjoyed working with his new aide. "The bathroom breaks aren't nearly as fun, though," he said.

"I bet," I replied. "Have you peed on the poor guy yet?"

Mike smiled. "No, I reserve that honor for very special people. I've never even peed on David."

"Let's keep it that way," David muttered. "I'd rather not receive that honor."

"How's the job?" Mike asked.

"Great! I am booked to deliver *The Money Game* seminar at various universities, and next month we are having a company meeting in Iowa. If you build it, they will come."

Mike looked into my eyes, and I could feel his hand on my shoulder. "Well," he said, "my little boy is all growns up."

My position with National Financial Educators proved stimulating and provided me with a solid income base. However, I like I had unfinished business. I missed Mike, and I wanted to do something for him – not by taking him to and from class, but on a larger scale. And one morning I figured out how.

Chapter 12

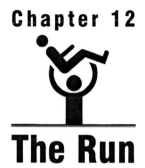

The Run

"Continuous, unflagging effort, persistence and determination
will win. Let not the man be discouraged who has these."
James Whitcomb Riley

Seven months later: April 2005

I love to run, but I never considered myself a runner. I didn't have the physical stamina or the mental willpower to endure more than a thirty minute jog. Nonetheless, I relished those 30 minutes early each morning, when the world was quiet and I was alone with my thoughts.

On the morning of April 1, 2005, my thoughts matched the weather – gloomy. As my breath quickened during my run, I thought of Mike. Mike.

Out of the gloom came a crazy idea. A zealous, perhaps foolish, daydream. Suddenly, my mind flooded with possibilities, not obstacles. My adrenaline soared, and my legs bounded, pumping faster and faster. I ran. Faster and longer than ever before.

As I approached Olmstead Street, my pace slowed to a walk as my thoughts continued to accelerate. My whole body shook with enthusiasm as I considered making my "dream" a reality. For a brief moment, I doubted. I wondered if this were fate's version of an April Fools prank: Inspire an out-of-shape dreamer into running 1,200 miles, and laugh as he stumbles after mile two. No. With every step I became more certain.

I would take Mike and David to Orlando for an unforgettable vacation—movies, shopping, and excitement at the mecca of magical thinking, Disney World. Then, I would embark on a run that would change my life forever.

As soon as I got home, I e-mailed long-distance runner Stu Mittleman and asked for his guidance. I knew that Stu had run a thousand miles in 11 days, and from San Diego to New York City. He replied to my e-mail within one day with his phone number. I called. He answered on the second ring. I explained my crazy idea. "That is a serious goal," he said. "Are you an accomplished runner?"

I cringed. "Not at all … but I believe anything is possible."

Stu agreed to be my coach, and over the next few days he sent me a diet plan and a strict training schedule. Four months hence, I would run from Orlando to Chicago. For Mike.

May 2005

After six weeks of phone calls, e-mails and an arduous training schedule, I was leaving for San Diego to run side by side with the greatest long-distance runner in the world, my mentor and coach, Stu.

As I awaited the call to board, I struggled to keep my legs from moving. Six weeks earlier, a three-mile run had exhausted me. Now, standing still required effort. Everyday running felt effortless. Second nature. I could not believe how much fun I was having; I actually enjoyed running. At the end of each run, I eagerly anticipated the next – the straining of my muscles, the fight to finish the last five minutes, the quickness of my breath, and the high upon completion.

The doubts that once plagued me had been crushed with every stride. I rejected all negative thoughts and fears. I would not let anything or anyone stop me – above all, myself. My confidence was soaring. My mind remained focused on the ultimate goal.

During my training with Stu, we scheduled the San Diego trip to gauge my progress. I considered the past six weeks my trial period wherein I had endeavored to prove my determination and grit to Stu. So I had run every day. When the training schedule demanded a 45-minute interval, I ran 65 minutes. I always strived for more. Always.

I felt more like a runner each day. I felt my body change and evolve, priming for 40 miles a day in the heat of the Deep South. My muscles strengthened, and my endurance improved. I felt physically powerful and, above all, healthy. By August, I intended to average eight to twelve hours a day. Tomorrow, I would run with Stu for five hours, longer than ever before. As I boarded the plane that Monday afternoon, I felt ready. I felt ready to conquer the world.

I awoke to the San Diego sun, brimming with anticipation. I waited for Stu impatiently, my legs eager to move, my body craving that runner's high.

Stu arrived at 9 a.m. bearing gifts – water, lotion, and Band-Aids. My coaching started immediately.

"Here." Stu extended the Band-Aids.

"For blisters?" I asked.

"No. For your nipples." He smiled. "Rookie."

With my nipples protected against chafing, Stu and I began with a brisk, fifteen-minute walk, as was the routine with my training. I wanted to break into a sprint, bolstered by the overwhelming thrill I felt in Stu's presence. I felt honored.

And then, finally, we ran.

We exchanged pleasantries – weather, sports, even a little celebrity gossip. I asked about long-distance running and his career. I longed to ask him a single question, one that I'd asked myself over and over on the plane, and again that morning as I waited.

"Stu…" I hesitated. "Why did you think I could do this?"

When I had contacted Stu, I could barely run more that two miles at one time. I could not comprehend why Stu agreed to train me with such eagerness and enthusiasm. I had no track record.

"That's easy, Tim," he responded. "Because you believe you can do it. That's all I needed. When people believe in themselves, they are astounded by what they can accomplish. This was no different. And working with you these past six weeks has only confirmed that – on many levels."

I was overwhelmed with pride. I'd earned Stu's respect. What an unforgettable moment – and lesson.

After two hours, we stopped by the beach to refill our water bottles. I breathed deeply, absorbing the fresh San Diego air and savoring the salty ocean breeze. I closed my eyes and listened to the crashing waves, to laughing children, and to my body. My limbs felt light and painless. My spirit soared. Stu's voice interrupted my reverie.

"Tim, you're doing great!" Stu exclaimed. "I'm impressed with your stamina. How do you feel?"

I smiled. "I feel great – like I can run forever!"

"Good ... 'cause we're going to keep on keeping on."

Clever, I thought, half smiling. *Don't quit your day job, Stu.*

We ran for three hours more. Our route extended along the shoreline, and through the city, past office buildings, sidewalk cafés and rowhomes. At times, we conversed about our lives and our goals, but mostly we ran in silence. Stu matched my pace. By the final hour, I could anticipate Stu's gait, and he mine. We conversed via running.

I realized something important that day. I've long known that success requires hard work – lots of hard work. After my conversations with Stu, I realized that faith in tandem with hard work is the catalyst for success. A belief in oneself makes any objective, however unattainable it might seem, achievable. With effort and steadfast faith in oneself, a janitor can become a CEO, a high school dropout can earn a Harvard degree, and a couch potato like me can become a long-distance runner.

Henry David Thoreau wrote: "If you have built castles in the air, your work need not be lost; that is where they should be. Now put the foundations under them." I'd set a lofty goal. For six weeks I'd been laying the foundations. I ran. Then, I ran some more. I believed in myself, and if not for that belief, my body would have shut down after week one. I'd built my castle in the sky, and soon I would reach it.

July 2005

The three-hour plane ride felt more like twenty-three hours as my mind raced with thoughts, from how to ensure an unforgettable vacation for Mike and David, to the logistics of the run. I felt scared, frustrated and anxious. Jason, our partner-in-crime in D.C., and my good friend Ryan were driving 20 hours straight from Chicago to Orlando. They had to arrive prior to my departure as Jason would accompany Mike and David home, while Ryan served as my driver on the first leg. My second driver, Justin, would arrive in Tallahassee a week later, and Dave, the driver for my longest and final leg would arrive in Atlanta a week thereafter. There was no room for error. No time to go off pace, get lost, or question myself. I had to run. Then I looked at Mike, strapped uncomfortably into his seat, and my nerves calmed as I remembered the reason behind it all.

Orlando was hot and muggy. We got to the hotel by noon and relished the air-conditioned room. It was a handicapped-accessible room, meaning the bathroom was larger and equipped with bars, none of which was useful to Mike. The room was littered with brochures, and Mike, David and I were eager to plan our day at the Magic Kingdom.

"Can we do *Pirates of the Caribbean*?" David asked excitedly. I located the attraction in the brochure. There was a disclaimer: Guests must transfer from a wheelchair to the attraction/ride vehicle. For safety and comfort, you should be in good health and free from heart, back or neck problems. Every attraction on Mike and David's list – Space Mountain, Splash Mountain, the Haunted Mansion – had the same disclaimer. Mike's eyes glazed over with disappointment.

"I'm sorry, little buddy," I said. I felt like an idiot. I'd thought of Disney World as the holy grail of adventures, when in reality the three of us could have driven north 60 miles to Kenosha, Wisconsin, and had just as much fun without reminding Mike of everything he couldn't do. I wanted to make Mike smile. I located the more accessible attractions in the brochure.

"Well," I said. "We could check out the 'foot-stompin', hand-clappin' musical revue performed by a band of backwoods bears and their furry friends!'"

Mike smiled. "Yeehaw."

"Or, we could travel to Cinderella's Castle, 'the formidable gateway to Fantasyland!'"

"Fantasyland?" David chimed in. "Will Pam Anderson be there?"

"Oh wait! This is the one! Tree trunk tunnels! Whimsical water fountains! And … wait for it … a honey pot! Let's go to Pooh's Playful Spot!"

In a deadpan tone, Mike said: "Why go to Pooh's spot? I have a poo right here in my pants." We couldn't stop laughing for the remainder of the trip.

As usual we made the best of it, spending most of our vacation at the Disney Marketplace, watching movies and shopping. The highlight of our adventure was meeting Pat Williams, founder and senior vice president of the Orlando Magic. In the weeks before the vacation, I contacted Pat through a mutual friend and requested a tour of the RDV Sportsplex where the Magic practiced. To my surprise and delight, Pat replied with an invitation. We were honored to receive a personal tour with one of America's top motivational and inspirational speakers and renowned authors.

As we left the complex, Pat pulled me aside.

"Tim, I'm touched by your relationship with Mike and David, and inspired by the great mission you are undertaking. I'm always inspired by people who take on something bigger than themselves."

"Wow. Thank you," I said, humbled. "Any advice?"

"Remember, if your *why* is big enough, facts don't matter." He paused. "And watch out for semis. Those guys really move!"

The next day, I stood at the on-ramp to Highway 90. My moment had arrived, and I was ready. I waved goodbye to Mike, and started running. The night before, we'd had dinner together at the Magic Kingdom, and now the time was here. I had rehearsed this in my mind a million times. Now it was real.

As I started running, I turned to see Mike disappearing into the distance. Ahead lay my long journey. I found myself awestruck by the vastness of human capability. For so long I had forced my body to the brink, and now I'd discovered its self-healing resiliency. Each day, I compelled my mind to accept unthinkable possibilities and realized its influential power.

With every stride, I tested my heart, physically and emotionally, and I discovered its immense strength. Four years earlier, I'd felt lost. And on one inspired morning, I'd become a man with a purpose. Each consecutive success reinforced my conviction. Mike is my inspiration.

A word from Stu Mittleman
Ultra-Distance World Champion, Author, Inspirational Speaker

My first encounter with Tim Wambach came, appropriately enough on April 1, 2005. He left me a voice mail message asking me if I would consider taking him on as a client because he wanted to run from Orlando to Chicago, later on that year. I kept listening to his message expecting it to end with: "Never mind, April's Fools!" Those words never appeared.

Far from it. Once we began to speak, I realized that this courageous and caring visionary was intent on making a difference in the life of another - in a very real and personal way. Tim's motivation was genuine and his fearlessness in leaving his comfort zone was both inspirational and irresistible. Of course I HAD to do all I could to support Tim; it was the least I could do in the presence of such of, what seemed to me at the time, an "heroic" and self less act.

When we started our work together, I had two questions for him: "Why" and "What's your running background?" Tim answered that he was so taken by the experience of "knowing" such a amazing person as Mike that he just could not hold back taking massive action to bring attention to the special "gifts" and "challenges" of those affected by Cerebral Palsy. His background then as a runner - oh my! - was basically non-existent.

Tim was a quick study with an insatiable thirst for personal growth and development. We met in person in San Diego, the following month, on May 16th, and ran together for 5 hours! That was the DOUBLE the amount he had ever previously run. Not that I ever doubted it from the moment we first talked, but then and there I knew for certain that whatever Tim set his mind to doing - he would accomplish.

Tim's gift originates in his motives that are pure and giving, born of friendship and love. From that "center", Tim adds his own very personal trait: His willingness to "go" where others might not dare. We all have much to learn from Tim, and Mike, and their journey together.

Stu Mittleman
Ultra-Distance World Champion, Author,
Inspirational Speaker

Afterword

When I was five, I wanted to be Batman – not because of some perverse fascination with tights, but to help others. In high school, I wanted to be a baseball player. Alas, one fateful day in my sophomore year, I hit a line drive down the left-field line and took off running. Spurred by adrenaline and enveloped in the moment, I passed first base, then second, but I did not hear the umpire call out, "Foul ball! Foul ball!" I rounded third and slid into home without being tagged. I looked at the umpire. He looked at me. "Foul ball," he said.

The fans were laughing, and I picked up my bat, determined to save face. I didn't. I proceeded to strike out. The fans laughed louder. It was the first time I'd felt vulnerable on a baseball field, and I never fully regained my confidence.

When I celebrated my 21st birthday, I had no idea what I wanted to be. One morning, while reading the sports page, I noticed an advertisement for a seminar titled *Unleash the Power Within: Fear Into Power,* hosted by Tony Robbins. I decided to attend, and as I watched Robbins command the stage and speak passionately about focus, physiology, and the Ultimate Success Formula, I felt inspired. I watched my fellow spectators absorb every word, and I heard story after story about how Robbins altered their lives for the better.

It was at that seminar that I discovered my calling – or rather, rediscovered my calling. I wanted to be Batman. I wanted to help people.

From that moment, I developed a thirst for the knowledge bestowed by Robbins and motivational speakers of his caliber. I read voraciously—Robbins, Jack Canfield, Og Mandino, Brian Tracy, Pat Williams, Dale Carnegie, and Napoleon Hill. It was in Hill's book *Think and Grow Rich* that I came upon the phrase "keep on keeping on." It resonated with me instantly, and it has been my motto ever since.

That was long before I was introduced to Mike, but those words never truly meant anything *until* I met Mike. Every second of his life, Mike embodies the concept of "keep on keeping on" his attitude, his perseverance, his outlook on life.

But in 2005, after my run from Florida to Chicago, I felt disappointed. The run did not generate, as I'd hoped, a widespread awareness of people with special needs. Nor was I any closer to my ambition of motivational speaking. To regain momentum, I decided to create a foundation called Keep On Keeping On.

Mike is the inspiration of the foundation. He moved me to want to help on a larger scale, and my friends and fellow founding members Dave Kunicki and Dan Joyce championed the cause as well. Immediately, we started devising ways to continue to raise awareness. We planned an annual Christmas fund-raiser called "Santa Cause" that has been wildly successful. Without Mike, none of us ever would have come together to start making a difference for the special needs community – in particular, for children born with cerebral palsy, muscular dystrophy, and other severe physical disabilities. Mike has that effect on people.

The overwhelmingly positive reaction to what we were trying to do proved to us that this was our calling. Armed with a dream and a call to action, we applied for and received 501(c)(3) tax status in August 2007, and the Keep On Keeping On Foundation (KOKO) was officially born. What started as three motivated individuals—Dave, Dan and myself—has already grown to a team of over 40 volunteers, all eager to make a difference in the lives of those in need.

We have formed a relationship with Pathways Center in Glenview, Ill., and have paid for many therapy sessions for kids who need it the most. We purchased a wheelchair for a child who outgrew his old one. We gave a family a machine that removes impurities in the air, providing a young man more oxygen and a better quality of life. We widened a doorway within a home, allowing another young man greater mobility and independence as he prepares for college. And, we donated funds toward making the playground at Welles Park in Chicago more handicapped accessible. These are just a few of the things we have been able to do with our organization. We want to do more.

The Keep On Keeping On Team (Team KOKO) consists of a group of caring volunteers eager to make a difference in the Chicago-land Special Needs Community. We are not unique because we help; we are unique in the ways that we help. Our annual "24-Hour Run" and "March Forth Banquet" are ways in which we generate much needed awareness for our cause. A main goal of ours at KOKO is to educate people about the difficulties of having a disability and to help them realize how much those afflicted with a handicap have to offer.

We understand the tendency of some to "look the other way" when they see someone in a wheelchair. We were once like them. We know that once people take the time to get to know these souls and appreciate what they go through, they will see what we now see. It will forever be our duty to help others to see more than just a "chair" or a disability.

KOKO is able to share the power of its message thanks to the support of its donors and volunteers. We welcome all levels of donation, whether it's a one-time gift or a monthly contribution. And we are always looking for motivated volunteers – people with high energy and a strong desire to make a difference in the world – to join our team. This is a rare opportunity to champion and help to mold a nonprofit organization in its beginning stages. For more information on donating or volunteering, visit www.KeepOnKeepingOn.org.

The story never ends. Life goes on, and we need people like Mike to remind us of all the amazing things human beings have to offer, whether they are disabled or not. We believe that anything is possible, and we will never give up on those who need our help most. We live by a simple motto: As long as you have a pulse, you must never give up – you must always keep on keeping on.

A word from David Kunicki
Executive Director, Keep On Keeping On Foundation

For far too long in my life, I felt a nagging emptiness – a feeling that what I was doing was meaningless, and that any goals I had were selfish and ultimately pointless. Deep down, I knew I wanted to make a difference and live with a purpose, but I didn't know how.

When I examined my life during these times, I would find comfort in the fact that I wasn't alone – not even close. I noticed most of my friends were the same way, working only for a paycheck and consumed by empty things like booze and sex. It was like I was a member of an army of zombies going through the motions of life. It was a dangerous place, a lonely place, but one that had safety in numbers.

This vacant life I was leading was coming to a head. So many bad decisions, usually caused or accompanied by alcohol, had led me to a crossroads. I knew one more selfish mistake could lead me past the point of no return.

It was at these crossroads that I bumped into Tim Wambach one afternoon in April 2005 at Wildwood Park on the northwest side of Chicago. Tim and I grew up together but had not spoken in the past several years. Tim caught me up, and he told me that he had decided to do something bold. And it was by Tim's inspiration that I decided to be bold as well and lift myself out of my zombie-like existence.

Tim told me he planned to run from Orlando to Chicago later that summer to raise awareness for cerebral palsy. It was the craziest thing that I had ever heard – and because of that, I told Tim: "I'm in, whatever you need!" I didn't hesitate because I knew that it would take something bold and it would take something a bit "crazy" – and most importantly, it would take something *real* – to shake me out of the funk I had been in for far too long and put me on a path that truly meant something.

I served as Tim's driver on the third leg of his run. During that time, Tim told me about his relationship with Mike, about how much Mike meant to him, and how he often wished he could trade places with him. For the first time, Tim helped me fully understand the definition of love. I realized that the power of Tim and Mike's friendship was exactly the feeling that was lacking in my life. While Tim had once led the same empty life I was leading, Tim ultimately found his meaning through Mike.

The momentum we gained from the run helped inspire us to create the Keep On Keeping On Foundation. While our defined goal is to specifically help those born with physical disabilities, what's equally important to me is our emphasis on celebrating anyone who has overcome life's obstacles. Starting in 2010, every March 4th we will honor some of these brave souls at our annual "March Forth Banquet."

Beating adversity, whether it be physical, mental or otherwise, is one of the great challenges of our human existence. It's what ultimately saved my life and gave it purpose. I hope that you can join us for "March Forth" and that it gives you the motivation to keep inspired, keep aware, and march forward past the struggles of your own life.

A word from Molly Mulcrone
Creative director, Handicap This Productions

In the early morning of April 18, 2008, a 5.2-level earthquake shook Chicagoland. Later that day, I received the first of many phone calls from Tim that rocked my little world. Mike and Tim had an idea.

"Mike and I want to take our educational outreach talks and turn them into a two-man show that we can take on the road. Mike was thinking it would be kind of like John Leguizamo's *Freak*, only with two guys. And on wheels," I said. "Literally."

"Yes!"

That was the day Handicap This Productions was conceived. Our mission is to work in conjunction with the Keep On Keeping On Foundation in raising awareness about people born with severe physical handicaps; to empower individuals to achieve their goals and dreams; and to further KOKO's mission with educational and entertaining performance art.

Our flagship project is the self-titled production *Handicap This*, which strings together a series of vignettes to highlight the incredible relationship between Mike and Tim. They happen to be natural entertainers, so the stage is the best medium for them to bring their story to life, share their journey, and educate people along the way. It also allows Mike to fulfill one of his many dreams – to make the crowd go wild!

While parts of this book are incorporated into the show, *Handicap This* does not duplicate it. It is a collage of moments, messages and humor that invite audiences to see Mike, not just his wheelchair. We hope that our shows will allow able-bodied people to see how they and handicapped people are alike, and that audiences will be inspired to pursue their dreams regardless of what obstacles they encounter.

Most of all, we'd like to break through the fear that causes people to avert their eyes when they see a handicapped person. Our goal is to educate the naïve, combat the spread of ignorance, and resurrect the humor that political correctness has suppressed. Mike is always the first to crack a joke about his handicap. What could be better than the magic of humor to disarm our resistance to what is different and learn to accept ourselves and one another?

Handicap This Productions goes still further to fulfill the Keep On Keeping On Foundation's mission in assisting individuals born with severe handicaps. Just as KOKO works with a family to expand the doorway to their home to let a wheelchair gain access, we are expanding Mike's doorway to life so that he can more easily access his dreams.

We hope Handicap This Productions will set the stage for others born with physical handicaps to showcase their talents, see their dreams realized, and keep on keeping on.

To find out more about us, visit our website at:
www.HandicapThis.com

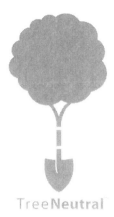

TreeNeutral

Advantage Media Group is proud to be a part of the Tree Neutral™ program. Tree Neutral offsets the number of trees consumed in the production and printing of this book by taking proactive steps such as planting trees in direct proportion to the number of trees used to print books. To learn more about Tree Neutral, please visit **www.treeneutral. com.** To learn more about Advantage Media Group's commitment to being a responsible steward of the environment, please visit **www. advantagefamily.com/green**

How We Roll is available in bulk quantities at special discounts for corporate, institutional, and educational purposes. To learn more about the special programs Advantage Media Group offers, please visit **www.KaizenUniversity.com** or call 1.866.775.1696.

Advantage Media Group is a leading publisher of business, motivation, and self-help authors. Do you have a manuscript or book idea that you would like to have considered for publication? Please visit **www.amgbook.com**

CPSIA information can be obtained at www.ICGtesting.com
Printed in the USA
LVOW131722030413

327366LV00002B/7/P